CELL BIOLOGY RESEARCH PROGRESS

# DYSPLASIA

## CAUSES, TYPES AND TREATMENT OPTIONS

# CELL BIOLOGY RESEARCH PROGRESS

Additional books in this series can be found on Nova's website under the Series tab.

Additional E-books in this series can be found on Nova's website under the E-books tab.

# PHYSIOLOGY - LABORATORY AND CLINICAL RESEARCH

Additional books in this series can be found on Nova's website under the Series tab.

Additional E-books in this series can be found on Nova's website under the E-books tab.

CELL BIOLOGY RESEARCH PROGRESS

# DYSPLASIA

## CAUSES, TYPES AND TREATMENT OPTIONS

LAUREL M. SEXTON
AND
HERSHEL J. LEACH
EDITORS

Nova Science Publishers, Inc.
*New York*

For permission to use material from this book please contact us:
Telephone 631-231-7269; Fax 631-231-8175
Web Site: http://www.novapublishers.com



**Library of Congress Cataloging-in-Publication Data**

Dysplasia : causes, types, and treatment options / editors, Laurel M. Sexton and Hershel J. Leach.
p. cm.
Includes index.
ISBN 978-1-61942-600-9 (hardcover)
1. Dysplasia. 2. Dysplasia--Diseases--Treatment. 3. Colon (Anatomy)--Diseases--Diagnosis. 4. Polyps (Pathology) I. Sexton, Laurel M. II. Leach, Hershel J.
RC280.C6D97 2011
617.5'547--dc23
2011049543

*Published by Nova Science Publishers, Inc. † New York*

# CONTENTS

# PREFACE

In this book, the authors present topical research in the study of the causes, types and treatment options for dysplasia. Topics discussed include colonic polyps and hereditary polyposis syndromes; developmental hip dysplasia; the causes and treatment options for bone dysplasia; a discussion on whether elevated intracellular chloride causes epilepsy in cortical dysplasia and dysplasia in ulcerative colitis.

Chapter 1 - Five percent of colorectal cancers are directly related to inherited genetic defects. Most of these tumors are diagnosed as pre-cancerous polyps. The purpose of this chapter is to identify the various colorectal pre-cancerous lesions, their natural history and their potential risks for malignancy. The clinical manifestations of Hereditary Polyposis Syndromes, Familial Adenomatous Polyposis, Gardner's Syndrome, and Turcot's Syndrome are discussed. Specific attention is drawn to Hereditary NonPolyposis Colorectal Carcinoma (HNPCC) with regard to Lynch I and Lynch II Syndromes. Specific gene mutations associated with increased risk for colorectal precursor lesions are inherently identified, with particular interest in mutations of the APC tumor suppressor and DNA mismatch repair genes.

The chapter highlights syndromes associated with colonic polyposis including Peutz-Jeghers Syndrome, and Juvenile Polyposis, while differentiating the malignant, sessile, adenomatous, villous polyps from their benign, pedunculated, hyperplastic, hamartomatous, tubular counterparts. The role of screening colonoscopy, sigmoidoscopy, Fecal Occult Blood Testing and Barium Enema in polyp detection and early cancer prevention is outlined.. Furthermore, an approach to various lesions based on age, genetic risk factors and family history, screening methods and histologic type is explained. This incorporates the indications for prophylactic surgery and periodic follow-up scoping. In conclusion, the authors summarize the guidelines to management with a unifying paragraph in relation to the aforementioned.

Chapter 2 - Developmental dysplasia of hip presents with a spectrum of disease. The natural history of it is poorly appreciated and for this reason, the exact role of various screening programmes and treatments is also poorly understood. Correspondingly, different nations have pursued differing strategies for treating infants with developmental dysplasia of hip.

In this chapter, the authors review the terminology to be aware of, the risk factors and various presentations of hip dysplasia as well as the importance of clinical examination and the role of imaging studies.

Screening is controversial and the authors rehearse the arguments for and against it. The authors also discuss the various treatments options available; these are dependent upon the age of presentation.

Chapter 3 - Bone dysplasias are a large and heterogeneous group of entities with a monogenic origin, cause changes in growth and bone development. Can be monostotic or polyostotic, affecting different areas of the bone and causing complications in the short, medium and long term. Molecular biology techniques allow prenatal diagnosis can be supported by imaging techniques in utero. Currently there are two classifications are used: a radiological classification, developed in 2001, which includes 33 groups of dysplasia and 3 groups of dysostosis based on the commitment of bone segments. So that the authors can find metaphyseal, diaphyseal and epiphyseal bone dysplasia according to the affected bone segment in long bones. Spondylo bone dysplasia if there is commitment of the spine. O bone dysplasias affecting specific bones as the skull or clavicles. And another molecular classification, basis of genetic alteration, which consists of several groups depending on whether the defect causing the disease is found in extracellular structural proteins, in metabolic pathways (ion channels, enzymes or transporters), in the folding and degradation of macromolecules or in the absence of proteoglycan degradation as in lysosomal diseases, in hormones or signal transduction mechanisms, in nuclear protein or transcription factors, in oncogenes and tumor suppressor genes or in metabolism and processing of DNA and RNA. Treatment options, as well as genetic counseling, are medical and surgical measures. They have no purpose but to support healing. In some types of bone dysplasia has recommended the use of bisphosphonates for prevention of vertebral fractures, remains controversial use of growth hormone.

Chapter 4 - γ-Aminobutyric acid (GABA) is the principal inhibitory neurotransmitter in the brain, and conventional anticonvulsant drugs often target the $GABA_A$ receptor chloride channel. However, GABA can become excitatory when intracellular chloride concentrations ($[Cl^-]_i$) are high. Depolarizing actions of GABA are seen not only in early development, but also in various pathological conditions. Cation-$Cl^-$cotransporters play critical roles in the regulation of $[Cl^-]_i$. Extrusion of $Cl^-$ from cells is achieved by $K^+$-$Cl^-$cotransporters (KCCs), whereas $Na^+$-$K^+$-$2Cl^-$cotransporters (NKCCs) promote intracellular accumulation of $Cl^-$. So far, at least four different mammalian subtypes of KCCs (KCC1-4) and two different subtypes of NKCCs (NKCC1-2) have been sequenced. Of these, KCC2 is present only in neurons while NKCC1 is expressed at moderate levels in both neurons and glial cells in the normal adult brain (Kanaka et al. 2001). In an animal model of epilepsy, NKCC1 expression has been found to be increased, while KCC2 mRNA was decreased in the hippocampus. Such changes in NKCC1 and/or KCC2 could lead to elevated $[Cl^-]_i$, and thereby cause an impairment in GABA-mediated inhibition. The authors have recently reported that KCC2 mRNA and protein levels were reduced in small neurons located around large abnormal neurons (giant cells) in human focal cortical dysplasia (FCD). However, NKCC1 expression did not differ among these cell types. These results indicate that downregulation of KCC2 may play a key role in the onset of seizures in FCD. Thus, high $[Cl^-]_i$ may play a role in inducing epilepsy in the human brain, through changes in $Cl^-$ regulation by KCC2 and NKCC1.

Chapter 5 - *Introduction:* patients with longstanding ulcerative colitis (LUC) have a high risk of developing colorectal cancer, compared to the general population. The highest risk appears in patients with extensive colitis, an intermediate risk in those having left-sided colitis whereas people with proctitis have practically no higher risk that the general population.

*Contents:* Dysplasia in UC is classified in low grade dysplasia, high grade dysplasia and indefinite for dysplasia, depending on the presence or absence of specific epithelial alterations. Protrusive lesions in UC are traditionally named DALMs (dysplasia associated lesion or mass). The degree of dysplasia is very important as it has an impact upon the sensitivity and specificity of the subsequent development of colorectal cancer. Dysplasia, irrespective of its grade, was reported to have a 74% sensitivity in the development of colorectal cancer, and in the same series studied in Mayo Clinic, high grade dysplasia had a smaller sensitivity (34%) but a 98% specificity in the detection of colorectal cancer. In a very recent meta-analysis, it was stated that the sensitivity of low grade dysplasia is associated with a 9 fold increase in the risk of developing colorectal cancer and a 12 fold increase in the risk of developing advanced neoplasia. It is therefore advisable to perform regular colonoscopic screening using different methods to detect dysplasia and/or early cancer. However this approach was not yet proved unequivocally to reduce mortality due to UC associated colorectal cancer. Beside simple colonoscopy, now there are new methods for colon surveillance: confocal chromoscopic endomicroscopy, chromoscopic colonoscopy, narrow band imaging (NBI), endoscopic trimodal imaging but these methods are not yet standardized. As treatment options, according to ECCO statements, high grade dysplasia in flat mucosa and adenocarcinoma are indications for proctocolectomy. A patient with low grade dysplasia in flat mucosa should be offered proctocolectomy or repeat surveillance biopsies within 3–6 months.

*Conclusion:* Since dysplastic changes of the colonic mucosa are associated with a high risk of colorectal cancer in patients with UC it is imperative to implement a colonoscopic surveillance program with the goal of reducing mortality and morbidity associated with colorectal cancer and in the same time to avoid unnecessary prophylactic colectomies, thus offering a less invasive treatment. Current strategies are difficult to keep, time consuming and expensive but apparently not effective enough to this purpose. Future efforts should be focused on a more accurate evaluation of individual risk factors for patient selection and an improvement of endoscopic techniques.

Chapter 6 - *Introduction:* Bronchial dysplasia is the most common premalignant lesion found in lung. In addition to other alterations, the authors have previously shown that in comparison to normal bronchial mucosa, bronchial dysplasia demonstrates increased vascular endothelial growth factor (VEGF) expression and increased angiogenic activity as measured by microvessel densities. The characterization of angiogenesis in bronchial dysplasia has been extended herein to include analysis of other angiogenic factors and to establish a mechanistic relationship between factor expression and angiogenic activity.

*Materials and Methods: In situ* characterization of angiogenic factor expression has been performed via quantitative RT-PCR on frozen tissue from 64 bronchial biopsies and 34 matched tumor-normal pairs. Epithelial cultures from bronchial biopsies representing a range of histologies have been used to study effects of conditioned media on endothelial cell proliferation, migration and tubulogenesis.

*Results:* Characterization of angiopoietin pathway factor expression shows that levels of angiopoietin-1, angiopoietin-2 and their receptor Tie2 are not different between bronchial dysplasia and normal bronchial epithelium, but are reduced in tumor tissue as compared to its matched normal tissue. Conditioned media from cultures of bronchial dysplasia shows induction of endothelial cell proliferation (5/6 dysplasia cell lines), migration (6/7) and tubule elongation (5/6) but no induction of new tubule formation (0/6). Addition of neutralizing anti-VEGF antibody completely abrogates proliferation, migration and tubule elongation induced by dysplasia derived conditioned media in nearly all cell lines tested.

*Conclusions:* Angiogenic activity in bronchial dysplasia appears to be largely mediated by VEGF. Although other factors may contribute to angiogenesis in bronchial dysplasia in some cases, this appears to be more prominent in invasive lung cancer. Features that distinguish angiogenic activity in bronchial dysplasia versus invasive lung cancer will be discussed. The potential interaction between angiopoietin and VEGF mediated angiogenesis in the development of lung cancer is explored. Distinct characteristics of bronchial dysplasia associated angiogenesis may have important implications in using these factors as markers of bronchial dysplasia or as targets for chemoprevention in lung cancer.

Chapter 7 - In the United States 350 000 people die yearly of SCD which does not spare any age, gender, or socioeconomic group. Major cause of SCD accounts for CAD, but smaller percentage is due to cardiac diseases other then CAD. The main substrate of latter are cardiac arrhythmias, mainly caused by ARVD/C, Long QT sy and WPW sy in those otherwise healthy population. Special problem exists in professional sports and dieing during sport activities, in spite being regularly thoroughly examined.

The most mysterious among aforementioned is arrhythogenic right ventricular dysplasia and/or cardiomyopathy (21 clinical genotype types) which unfortunately, apparently, has no clinical warning sign at the early stage, sometimes having SCD for the first and only presenting dramatic event. The arrhythmias leading to SCD may be identified by electrophysiological testing, and significant percentage of patients can have polymorphic VT or VF as the only inducible arrhythmia, which seems to be the exact scenario for fatal outcome in the whole group of patients. So what might be the underlying cause and could it be prevented?

ARVD/C is genetically inherited condition with autosomal-dominant pattern of inheritance (as most common), as consequence of single gene mutations witch lead to complex patterns of altered localization of desmosomal proteins. These mutations may change cytosolic pools of cell-cell junction proteins which lead to desmosome disorganization and gap junction distortion. Latter is explanation for loss of contact between cardiomyocites and earlier start of apoptosis.

Pathological hallmark of ARVD/C is the atrophy of myocites with fatty or fibro-fatty infiltration of the right ventricle. Typical clinical picture encompasses arrhythmias with left bundle branch block morphology and ventricular tachyarrhythmias, while less frequent presentation are signs of right heart failure (fatigue and shortness of breath). Disease may be localized or widespread, with biventricular involvement in some cases.

Valid WHO criteria during last 12 years failed to detect disease at its early stage and recommended diagnostic methods were shown to have low sensitivity for majority of patients even in its overt phase (because of lack of scoring system). Investigation of this population is further complicated by disease rarity and lack of large databases. New research published data give priority to vectorcardiography and ultrasound.

The possible explanation for this lies in the existence of specific place in the heart exposed to most physical forces during cardiac cycle. Nevertheless, this place is *locus minoris rezistentio* during contraction and relaxation of the heart. It is presently focus of ongoing clinical study regarding two aforementioned methods in detecting early stage of ARVD/C. It is also registered by WIPO as SOPHIE methodology (suggesting wisdom to detect). Soon enough the authors can expect this technique to be incorporated in newly medical equipment (for stratification of risk for SCD).

In: Dysplasia
Editors: L. M. Sexton and H. J. Leach
ISBN 978-1-61942-600-9


*Chapter I*

# COLONIC POLYPS AND HEREDITARY POLYPOSIS SYNDROMES

***Viplove Senadhi*[1] *and Dennis Emuron*[2]**
[1]Division of Gastroenterology and Hepatology,
Brater Scholar, Indiana Institute for Personalized Medicine,
Division of Clinical Pharmacology,
Indiana University School of Medicine, US
[2]Johns Hopkins University/Sinai Hospital Program in Internal Medicine,
Sinai Hospital, Baltimore, MD, US

## ABSTRACT

Five percent of colorectal cancers are directly related to inherited genetic defects. Most of these tumors are diagnosed as pre-cancerous polyps. The purpose of this chapter is to identify the various colorectal pre-cancerous lesions, their natural history and their potential risks for malignancy. The clinical manifestations of Hereditary Polyposis Syndromes, Familial Adenomatous Polyposis, Gardner's Syndrome, and Turcot's Syndrome are discussed. Specific attention is drawn to Hereditary NonPolyposis Colorectal Carcinoma (HNPCC) with regard to Lynch I and Lynch II Syndromes. Specific gene mutations associated with increased risk for colorectal precursor lesions are inherently identified, with particular interest in mutations of the APC tumor suppressor and DNA mismatch repair genes.

The chapter highlights syndromes associated with colonic polyposis including Peutz-Jeghers Syndrome, and Juvenile Polyposis, while differentiating the malignant, sessile, adenomatous, villous polyps from their benign, pedunculated, hyperplastic, hamartomatous, tubular counterparts. The role of screening colonoscopy, sigmoidoscopy, Fecal Occult Blood Testing and Barium Enema in polyp detection and early cancer prevention is outlined.. Furthermore, an approach to various lesions based on age, genetic risk factors and family history, screening methods and histologic type is explained. This incorporates the indications for prophylactic surgery and periodic follow-up scoping. In conclusion, we summarize the guidelines to management with a unifying paragraph in relation to the aforementioned.

## Introduction

Colorectal cancer is the third most common cancer in the United States following cancer of the breast and lung, and is a major cause of cancer-related morbidity and mortality in North America and Europe. The bulk of evidence suggests that most colonic cancers arise within previously benign adenomatous polyps, which are precursor lesions for colorectal cancer. Adenomas are simply defined as benign tumors of glandular origin and are referred to as polyps if they project outward from the mucous membrane of the colon [1]. Inherent in the definition of colonic adenomas is that have undergone dysplasia.

Colorectal cancers can be categorized into hereditary (familial) and nonhereditary (sporadic) types; however, all cancers are assumed to have a genetic component that may be inherited or acquired to a varying degree. Individuals born into families with a history of hereditary colon cancer might have an altered genome that, with exposure to environmental factors, may progress to a malignant phenotype. Traditional genetic-environmental interactions contribute to the pathogenesis and to the multiple somatic mutations identified with nonhereditary cancers. The aforementioned is the classic "two hit" model of nature and nurture. For a schematic understanding of genetic pathogenesis, it can also be simplified into a second "two hit genetic model", where either a genetic pathway in tumor initiation ("first hit") or progression ("second hit") is disrupted. In Familial Adenomatous Polyposis, tumor initiation is accelerated, through loss of the APC gene. In contrast, in Hereditary NonPolyposis Colorectal Cancer, tumor progression is accelerated through loss of DNA Mismatch Repair (MMR) genes such as MLH1 and MSH2 [2]. Sporadic adenomas do not have accelerated pathways in either initiation or progression, but rather need both "hits" that take place from both environmental and other genetic factors such as loss K-ras oncogene mutations.

The role of genetics in the development of colon cancer is manifested in Hereditary Polyposis Syndromes. These syndromes are characterized by the presence of multiple polypoid lesions throughout the gastrointestinal tract - Polyposis, with or without extracolonic tumors. Hereditary Nonpolyposis Colorectal Carcinoma (HNPCC) is another inherited variant in which colon cancers arise in discrete adenomas in the absence of polyposis. Although colorectal cancer syndromes with apparent patterns of inheritance currently account for only a small percentage of total colorectal cancer cases, hereditary factors may be present in a large proportion of cases. Genetic susceptibility to colorectal cancer in the general population is suggested by the two to three-fold increase in colorectal cancer in the first-degree relatives of patients with sporadic adenomas and colorectal cancer, the relative risk being even stronger when cancer occurs in family members younger than 50 years of age. This has been taken into account in screening guidelines that stratify patients according to potential cancer risk. In this chapter, we will discuss the principle premalignant colonic lesions, which is the adenomatous polyps. We will examine adenoma distribution, predisposing factors to the development of colorectal adenomas and subsequent cancer, the clinical presentation of adenomas, the diagnosis, screening, management, and follow-up involved in detecting these precursor lesions.

## EPIDEMIOLOGY

The inherent risk for colon cancer in a population and the age of the subjects affect the prevalence of adenomatous polyps. Although the frequency of colonic adenomas is widely variant among populations, they are more frequent in populations at greater risk for colon cancer [3]. Adenoma prevalence also correlates with socioeconomic status even in regions of low colon cancer risk; however, this observation may be biased in favor of increased adenoma detection among those who can afford health care. Age is the single most important independent determinant of adenoma prevalence [4,5,6]. Multiple studies correlate age with a greater likelihood of large adenomas, multiple polyps and severely dysplastic adenomas. One half to two thirds of people over age 65 in high risk areas may harbor colonic adenomas [7,8]. Furthermore, the development of adenomas is independent of sex, although some studies of asymptomatic individuals from both autopsy [9] and colonoscopic [10] series have suggested that adenoma prevalence is higher in men. Race is not an independent determinant of developing colorectal adenomas [11].

## Risk Factors

Predisposing factors to developing colorectal adenomas and subsequent cancer include age, diet, personal history and family history. These factors interact at various levels to impede or promote malignant transformation. We will discuss diet and personal history, with more emphasis on family history as a significant factor.

## Diet

Colon cancer rates are comparatively higher in populations with high total fat intake in contrast to those consuming less fat [12,13]. Dietary fat is proposed to enhance cholesterol and bile acid synthesis by the liver thereby increasing amounts of these sterols in the colon. These lipid and sterol metabolites damage the colonic mucosa and increase the proliferative activity of the epithelium, promoting tumorigenesis.

Although the protective role of dietary fiber is not fully known, epidemiologic studies correlate high fiber intake with lower incidence of colon cancer [14,15]. Fermentation of fiber components by fecal flora to short-chain fatty acids decreases colonic pH and potentially inhibits carcinogenesis [16]. Circumstantial evidence also suggests a possible role for dietary calcium in prevention of colorectal cancer.

Dietary calcium binds to ionized fatty acids and bile acids in the gastrointestinal tract, converting them into insoluble, non-toxic calcium compounds. Because most colon cancers develop from adenomas, it is reasonable to expect that similar dietary factors would influence adenoma formation or progression. Alcohol consumption, especially beer, has been associated with an increased risk of rectal, but not colonic cancer [17,18].

However, one study found no correlation between alcohol consumption and either rectal or colonic adenomas [19]. Moreover, in another study, an apparent association between alcohol intake and distal colorectal adenomas disappeared after data was adjusted for dietary fat and fiber consumption [20]. Unfortunately, dietary modifications have not been validated in prospective interventional studies [21].

## Personal History

Preexisting history of colorectal adenomas and carcinomas are predisposing factors to colorectal cancer. The majority of colorectal cancers arise from pre-existing adenomas, the risk rising as the number of adenomas increases [22,23]. As adenomas grow, they progressively differentiate, become dysplastic and then become malignant [24]. Despite the potential for adenomas to undergo malignant change, the actual risk is unknown. The malignancy rate is higher in large adenomas, with villous architecture, cytologic nuclear atypia or dysplasia [25]. Individuals with one colorectal carcinoma have an increased risk of developing a second cancer either simultaneously (synchronous carcinomas) or subsequently (metachronous carcinomas).

## Family History

The risk of colorectal cancer in first degree relatives of those with sporadic colorectal cancer may increase three-fold. The role of family history in hereditary polyposis syndromes is discussed individually.

## Hereditary Polyposis Syndromes

Hereditary polyposis syndromes may be classified into familial or nonfamilial groups. Familial polyposis syndromes are histologically categorized into adenomas (polyps are true neoplasms) or hamartomas (polyps are not true neoplasms). Nonfamilial groups; cronkhite-canada syndrome [26], lymphoid polyposis [27], pseudopolyps, lipomatous polyposis, pneumatosis cystoides intestinalis are a heterogeneous collection of syndromes linked only by the presence of gastrointestinal polyps, and are not associated with an increased risk of cancer.

## Inherited Adenomatous Polyposis Syndromes

Inherited adenomatous polyposis syndromes include several entities that are characterized by the development of large numbers of adenomatous polyps in the colon. Familial polyposis coli and its variants which include Gardner's syndrome, attenuated familial adenomatous polyposis (AFAP) and many cases of Turcot's syndrome are inherited in an autosomal dominant fashion, and ultimately affected individuals with polyps eventually develop carcinoma in the absence of colectomy.

## Other Inherited Adenomatous Syndromes

Colorectal cancer is also associated with Hereditary Nonpolyposis colorectal cancer, Torre's or Muir's Syndrome, Peutz-Jeghers Syndrome and the familial form of Juvenile Polyposis, with cancers appearing to arise in adenomatous polyps. The various syndromes are distinguished by the presence or absence of extracolonic manifestations.

### Familial Adenomatous Polyposis (FAP)

#### *Genetics*

FAP is the most common adenomatous polyposis syndrome and is inherited as an autosomal dominant disease with 80% to 100% penetrance. Genetic mapping and restriction fragment length polymorphism (RFLP) analysis localizes gene responsible for FAP on chromosome 5q [28]. In addition, RFLP analysis suggests that the FAP locus might encode for a tumor suppressor gene with evidence of its loss, leading to tumor progression [29]. Approximately twenty percent of cases have a negative family history and represent new mutations at the adenomatous polyposis coli (APC) locus [30,31,32]. Germ line mutations associated with more extensive colon involvement manifesting as "colonic carpeting" are located in a 214-base pair sequence of the APC gene between codons 1250 and 1464, mutations elsewhere in the gene result in fewer colorectal polyps [33]. It is thought that it takes the loss of two APC alleles to cause development of adenomas. A germline mutation from the affected parent occurs initially and the second allele is lost sporadically. RFLP analysis has proven that sporadic adenomas are known to share this feature when they lose one of the alleles at the APC locus [34].

***Clinical Features***

FAP is characterized by the progressive development of hundreds of thousands of adenomatous polyps in the large intestine with inevitable development of colon cancer if not resected. In patients with FAP, the colonic mucosa is carpeted by hundreds to thousands of adenomatous polyps. These polyps are usually located in the proximal colon and tend to be flat growths due to intramural rather than intraluminal growth [35]. Following inheritance of the gene for FAP, patients are usually asymptomatic until puberty, where polyps may begin to appear; rarely, however, polyps appear in the first decade of life. An early series of FAP cases showed the average age at onset of polyps was 25 years with symptoms appearing at age 33 years. The average age for the diagnosis of adenoma was 36 years, for cancer 39 years and for death from cancer, 42 years. Ninety percent of FAP cases have been diagnosed by the time the patient is 50 years of age [36]. A study focusing on early screening reported that fifty percent of FAP gene carriers will have polyps at sigmoidoscopy by approximately age 15 [37]. The disease begins in younger patients with a small number of polyps, which progressively increases until the colon becomes studded with adenomas throughout its length. Tubular, tubulovillous, and villous adenomas may all be seen. The macroscopic number of polyps in a colectomy specimen averages 1000, but may be tens of thousands. Polyps tend to be more numerous in the symptomatic than asymptomatic populations discovered by screening, the vast majority being small (less than 5 mm). Colorectal cancer should be considered an inevitable consequence in the natural history of FAP, appearing approximately 10 to 15 years after the onset of the polyposis. Metastatic colorectal carcinoma is the most common cause of death in FAP patients. Colorectal cancer is found in seventy-nine percent of the index cases of FAP, but in only nine percent of asymptomatic relatives screened for the disease. Additionally, FAP patients tend to have multiple simultaneous cancers versus the general population [38]. Genetic markers and RFLP analysis can aid in the identification of gene carriers who have not yet developed polyps [39].

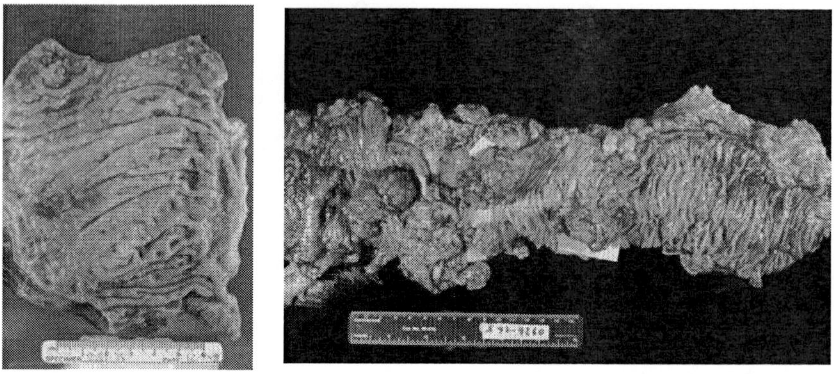

Figure 1. Familial adenomatous polyposis and polyposis occurring with carcinoma.

## Figures Demonstrating FAP

### *Extracolonic Involvement in FAP*

Lesions previously assumed to characterize Gardner's syndrome are recognized in many cases of FAP with various extracolonic site involvement.

### *Osteomas*

Bone abnormalities include osteomas of the mandible, skull, and long bones. Mandibular osteomas can be seen in up to ninety percent of patients with FAP. Osteomas can occur in children in the absence of colonic polyposis. Osteomas are usually multiple and can be diagnosed on plain x-rays and are usually removed if symptomatic or disfiguring.

### *Gastric and Duodenal Adenomas*

Polyps are present in the upper GI tract in nearly all FAP patients. Gastric polyps are almost universal in FAP patients and are most commonly of fundic gland origin. These particular fundic gland polyps grow in the absence of Proton Pump Inhibitors (PPI's), which are classically associated with fundic gland polyps. Unlike fundic gland polyps from PPI's, patients with FAP have epithelial dysplasia and require examination if of larger size, or in the presence of duodenal polyposis. Adenomatous polyps may also be found in the gastric antrum, duodenum, jejunum, ileum and periampullary region, which is the most commonly involved area [41,42,43]. In fact, many patients manifest with pancreatitis, due the adenomatous changes that take place at the Ampulla of Vater. The relative risk of duodenal cancer is markedly increased in patients with FAP or Gardner's syndrome, but no statistically significant increase in the risk for gastric or nonduodenal intestinal cancer has been documented [44]. In fact, the most common cause of death in patients with FAP after prophylactic colectomy is surprisingly from Duodenal cancer. Duodenal cancer increases with age and the incidence is close to 75%. The Spigelman Classification for Duodenal lesions classifyies relative risk. Jejunal and Ileal lesions tend to also occur, but are much less likely to be malignant. Fortunately, novel methods such as spiral enteroscopy and double balloon enteroscopy have been developed to achieve complete enteroscopy, which is required for surveillance.

### *Desmoid Tumors*

Diffuse mesenteric fibromatosis (Desmoid tumors) may complicate adenomatous polyposis syndromes and although they occur in approximately twenty percent of patients, they are the second most common cause of death after metastatic colonic carcinoma. Desmoids lead to gastrointestinal obstruction, constrict arteries, veins or ureters, and are associated with a 10% to 50% mortality rate. Desmoids tend to cluster in families in FAP patients, which warrants abdominal imaging in those individuals with a strong family history. Desmoids are also more common when the disease codon is distal to the codon 1444. Desmoid prediction and understanding is critical to the overall management of FAP patients, as desmoids most often appear after early colectomy especially in female patients. This feature has led some groups to advocate for delaying colectomy in this cohort of the population [45]. Radiation therapy though effective for localized desmoid tumors [46], is often impractical. Sulindac causes partial tumor shrinkage in some patients and a combination with tamoxifen is commonly used [47]. Patients with early stage disease may have a delayed colectomy-to-desmoid interval with a much better prognosis. Stage III and IV disease require chemotherapy [48], and a small bowel transplant should be considered in severe mesenteric disease.

### *Other Tumors*

Other soft tissue tumors have been described in FAP, which include epidermoid cysts, lipomas and fibromas. Multiple epidermal cysts may present prior to the diagnosis of FAP and FAP variants and clinical suspicion for Gardner's must be high in this setting.

## Gardner's Syndrome (A FAP Variant)

Gardner's syndrome, like Turcot syndrome, attenuated Familial Adenomatous Polyposis is a variant of FAP.

### *Genetics*

Gardner's syndrome is inherited as an autosomal dominant disease linked to the APC gene. Both are variable manifestations of a disease traced to a single genetic locus. Germ line mutations are found in patients with these two entities, and in most instances, the mutations created a stop codon which prevents successful transcription and translation. The biologic basis of the variable expression of these diseases is unknown.

### *Clinical Features*

Gardner's syndrome is a familial disease consisting of gastrointestinal polyposis predominantly involving the colon. The genetic, pathologic, and clinical characteristics of this disease include all of the features of FAP, expressing itself variably in different individuals within a single family, including skipped generations and discordance in identical twins [49].

The small intestine is subject to neoplastic growth in Gardner's syndrome as in FAP. The frequency of adenomatous polyposis and subsequent carcinoma in the periampullary region of the duodenum may be as high as 12 per cent [50].

Pancreatitis can develop from neoplasms of the papilla obstructing the pancreatic or biliary drainage system [51,52]. Small intestinal carcinoma outside the duodenum is rare. Multiple polyps including adenomas, fundic gland hyperplasia and microcarcinoids are found in the stomach [53], with gastric carcinoma as a rare complication of Gardner's syndrome in the western world [54,55].

The extracolonic manifestations of Gardner's syndrome include osteomas of the mandible, skull and long bones; dental abnormalities; exostoses; inclusion cysts; fibromas; lipomas; and biliary tree [56], liver, [57,58] adrenals [59] and thyroid [60] neoplasms. Second to metastatic carcinoma, desmoid tumors are among the lethal complications of Gardner's syndrome affecting approximately 8 to 13 per cent of patients [61,62]. Like some families with FAP, Gardner's syndrome may be characterized by Congenital hypertrophy of the retinal pigmented epithelium (CHRPE) [63]. These pigmented lesions of the ocular fundus may occur in ninety percent of cases with Gardner's syndrome [64].

## Turcot's Syndrome

### *Genetics*

Turcot's syndrome is defined by the association of familial colonic polyposis with malignant brain tumors [65]. Cerebellar Medulloblastomas and Glioblastoma Multiforme (GBM) are the brain tumors that are involved. Interestingly, GBM is more consistent with a HNPCC variant and is associated with a MMR gene defect. On the other hand, most patients with Turcot's syndrome that have developed Cerebellar Medulloblastomas, result from a germline APC mutation that is 90 times more likely in FAP patients. Thus, Turcot's can also be considered as a variant of FAP.

### *Clinical Features*

Features suggestive of a diagnosis of Turcot's syndrome include the presence of colonic polyposis and a malignant brain tumor like glioblastoma multiforme in a young person, or the presence of polyposis and brain tumors in siblings, but not in the parents.

This latter feature is a further reflection of the reputed autosomal recessive inheritance in Turcot's syndrome [66,67]. The patients tend to have fewer polyps than is typical of FAP [68].

## Muir's or Torre's Syndrome

### *Genetics*

These familial syndromes have a high incidence of colonic cancer associated with a small number of colonic adenomas and are probably part of the spectrum of HNPCC, [69] and are not to be confused with FAP or Gardner's syndrome.

### *Clinical features*

This syndrome manifests with sebaceous adenomas and carcinomas, basal cell and squamous cell carcinomas, keratoacanthomas, together with adenomas and adenocarcinomas of the colon [70].

# INHERITED HAMARTOMATOUS POLYPOSIS SYNDROMES

These syndromes are characterized by multiple hamartomatous polyps of the GI tract. Peutz-Jegher's syndrome and juvenile polyposis have been known to have documented cases of GI cancer develop, unlike their counterparts, von Recklinghausen's syndrome, [71] cowden's syndrome, [72] and basal cell nevus syndrome [73], that are not the scope of this chapter.

## Peutz-Jegher's Syndrome

### *Genetics*

This syndrome appears to follow an autosomal dominant pattern of inheritance with variable and incomplete penetrance [74,75].

### *Clinical Features*

The gene for Peutz-Jeghers syndrome confers an increased risk for GI and extraintestinal malignancies. This syndrome is characterized by mucocutaneous pigmentation most commonly around the nose, mouth, lips, buccal mucosa, hands, feet, perianal and genital sites that may be identified in early infancy. These melanin deposits tend to fade at puberty except for the buccal pigmentation. Polyps may be found in the stomach, small intestines or colon. Intestinal polyps may cause obstruction or intussusception which may occur as early as infancy [76]. Acute and chronic GI bleeding may complicate the disease. Foci of adenomatous epithelium may arise within the Peutz-Jeghers polyps, and these have been reported to develop into colon, duodenal, jejunal, and ileal carcinomas [77,78]. Ovarian cysts and tumors [79], and sertoli cell testicular tumors [80], pancreatic cancers [81], gallbladder and biliary tree polyps or cancers, [82] may occur in patients with Peutz-Jeghers syndrome. The diagnosis is usually made in the second decade, but the diagnosis of cancer is usually made in midlife prior to the age of 50. There is over a ninety precent risk in Peutz-Jegher's of developing cancer. Patients with this syndrome are at risk of cancer throughout the gastrointestinal tract and other organs including stomach, small bowel, pancreas, colon, breast and ovaries [83].

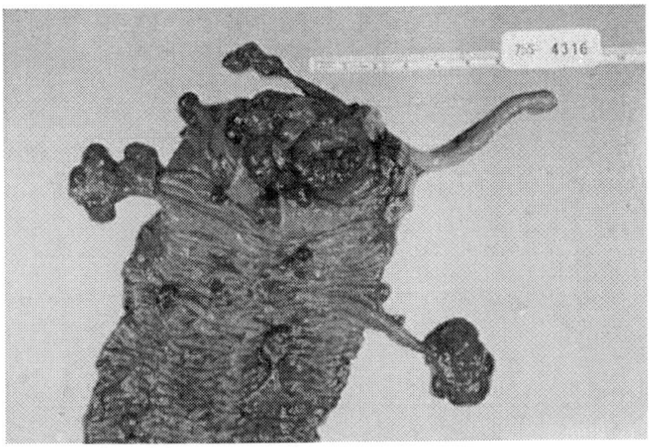

Figure 2. Gross pathologic demonstration of colonic Juvenile polyps.

## Juvenile Polyposis

### *Genetics*

This syndrome is inherited in an autosomal dominant fashion with some cases having multiple germ line mutations and others being sporadic.

### *Clinical Features*

Juvenile polyposis syndrome can be defined by any one of the following criteria; five or more juvenile polyps of the rectum or colon, juvenile polyps throughout the gastrointestinal tract, or any number of juvenile polyps in the gastrointestinal tract with a family history of juvenile polyps [84]. Contrary to the adenomatous syndromes that more than often present after puberty, Juvenile polyps produce symptoms in childhood typically presenting with gastrointestinal bleeding, obstruction and intussusception. There is increased risk of colon cancer with familial juvenile polyposis [85].

# Hereditary Nonpolposis Colorectal Carcinoma

Hereditary nonpolyposis colorectal carcinoma (HNPCC) is any collection of familial colorectal cancers exhibiting a mendelian form of inheritance exclusive of the adenomatosis coli syndromes. A number of families have shown a high incidence of adenocarcinoma of the colon in the absence of extensive colonic polyps [86]. These include Lynch syndrome I (HNPCC type a) and Lynch syndrome II (HNPCC type b).

## Genetics

Hereditary colorectal nonpolyposis coli is characterized by an autosomal dominant mode of genetic inheritance, and is a consequence of defective DNA mismatch repair. Cell-mediated immunologic defects might interfere with the recognition and killing of incipient tumor cells [87]. Genetic analysis localizes the Lynch syndrome II gene to chromosome 18 [88].

## Clinical Features

These carcinomas usually appear in the 40 to 50 year old patient group. Lynch I syndrome, site-specific HNPCC, includes families in which heritable cancer is limited to the colon and rectum, family members are also prone to cancers of the female genital tract and other anatomic sites. Patients with Lynch II syndrome like Lynch I have discrete polyps without polyposis which may precede carcinoma [89]. HNPCC tends to affect the proximal colon, in the presence of multiple primary malignancies with mucinous carcinoma as predominant histology [90].

# Conditions Associated with Adenomatous Polyps

Patients with acromegaly, streptococcus bovis bacteremia and those post ureterosigmoidoscopy have a strong predisposition to develop adenomatous polyps. Patients with breast cancer, skin tags, post cholecystectomy, atherosclerosis and cholesterol have documented associations with adenomatous polyps, but risk is not strong enough to recommend a surveillance policy.

## Acromegaly

Patients with acromegaly have increased tendency to develop adenomas and colon cancers [91,92]. Acromegalics with a family history of colon cancer [93] and those with multiple skin tags [94] have a higher risk for colonic neoplasia.

The mechanism of colonic neoplasia is not directly correlated to growth hormone levels [95] as the risk of neoplasia may even be greater in cured acromegalics compared to those with active disease. However, high serum IGF-1 levels have been correlated with increased epithelial cell proliferation [96] and increased recurrence rates of colorectal adenomas [97].

## Streptococcus Bovis Bacteremia

Bacteremia and endocarditis caused by S. bovis have been associated with adenomatous polyps [98], familial polyposis coli, [99] and colorectal carcinoma [100]. Patients with S. bovis bacteremia should undergo thorough colonic examination to exclude a malignancy.

## Ureterosigmoidostomy

Adenomatous polyps and carcinomas [101], juvenile polyps and inflammatory polyps are known to develop at ureterosigmoidostomy sites [102].

*N*-nitrosamines are thought to be generated from urinary amines in the presence of fecal flora with subsequent formation of the aforementioned lesions [103].

## Atherosclerosis and Cholesterol

Various autopsy studies have showed an association between adenomatous polyps and atherosclerosis [104,105]. However, no correlation between serum cholesterol levels and adenomatous polyps has been determined.

It goes without mentioning that the gene for two enzymes involved in cholesterol synthesis are located on chromosome 5, the same locus as the APC gene [106].

## Cholecystectomy

Cholecystectomy has been associated with a modest increase in risk for colon cancer, mainly occurring in women and the proximal colon [107]. In the absence of the gall bladder, it is hypothesized that increased delivery of bile acids enhances the proliferative activity of the colonic mucosa [108].

# Diagnosis and Screening

## Diagnosis

### *Signs And Symptoms*

History and physical examination are essential to diagnosis. However, most patients with colonic polyps may have nonspecific intestinal symptoms. Occult or overt rectal bleeding is the most common presentation attributed to colonic polyps. Because adenomas generally tend to maintain the integrity of the surface epithelium and may bleed into the polyp stroma [109,110], bleeding from polyps is more than often intermittent and does not usually cause fecal occult blood loss or anemia. Other symptoms include constipation, diarrhea, and flatulence. Constipation or decreased stool caliber is more likely due to bulky lesions in the distal colon. Cramping lower abdominal pain due to intermittent intussusception may also occur with large colonic polyps. Villous adenomas are occasionally associated with a syndrome of secretory diarrhea characterized by considerable and sometimes life-threatening water and electrolyte depletion, with dehydration, hyponatremia, hypochloremia, hypokalemia and metabolic acidosis [111]. Secretory villous adenomas exhibit a net secretion of water and sodium and an exaggerated secretion of potassium [112].

### *Investigation*

Colorectal polyps are typically detected in asymptomatic individuals being screened for colorectal neoplasia or incidentally during investigation for symptoms apparently referable to the colon. Polyps are occasionally diagnosed during specific workup for unexplained iron deficiency anemia.

***Fecal Occult Blood Testing (FOBT)***

In general, polyps under 1 cm in size do not bleed. Less than ten percent of people who report frank rectal bleeding will be found to have carcinoma *in situ*, an adenoma $\geq$ 1 cm [13,114]. Adenomas larger than 1.5 to 2.0 cm lose more than the usual amount of blood regardless of their location within the colon [115,116]. Only twenty to forty percent of patients with known adenomas show positive hemoccult test results [117,118], the rates being higher in patients with larger and distal polyps.

***Sigmoidoscopy***

Flexible fiberoptic sigmoidoscopy is three times superior to rigid sigmoidoscopy in detecting polyps (and cancer) in both symptomatic and asymptomatic patients [119]. The increased yield in detection is due primarily to the fact that 44 to 82 percent of polyps detected are located beyond the average depth of insertion of the rigid endoscope. [120,121,122]. The shorter 35-cm flexible sigmoidoscope compares favorably with the 60-cm flexible instrument for both colorectal neoplasm detection and patient acceptance [123,124].

***Barium Enema***

Double-contrast barium enema maximizes detection of small polyps while large polyps are readily detected by either the single-contrast or double-contrast enema [125,126]. Common sources of diagnostic error include inadequate colon preparation, and diagnostic difficulty in the presence of diverticulosis or redundant bowel.

***Colonscopy***

Colonoscopy is the gold standard for adenoma detection due to enhanced diagnostic accuracy and therapeutic capacity. This diagnostic superiority is demonstrated in various studies of patients with known polyps [127,128] and in symptomatic patients with inconclusive proctosigmoidoscopic and barium enema examinations. [129,130].

However, colonoscopy has some limitations that include failure to reach the cecum in about ten percent of cases; neoplasms located behind folds or at flexures could be missed; it requires patient sedation; and costs higher than barium enema.

### *Endoscope-Compatible Optic Fiber Systems*

This can be used to obtain laser-induced fluorescence spectra of mucosal abnormalities during endoscopy in real time. The spectrum emitted by adenomatous polyps is distinct from that of hyperplastic polyps and normal mucosa.

It appears most efficacious and safe for surveillance of the rectal stump in patients with familial polyposis coli following subtotal colectomy with ileorectal anastomosis [131].

## Screening

Cancer prevention is categorically primary or secondary. Primary prevention entails identifying the etiologic genetic, biologic and environmental factors and averting their effects on carcinogenesis. Secondary prevention identifies existing preneoplastic and early neoplastic lesions whether symptomatic or not, and managing them expeditiously. The two main approaches to colon cancer screening are fecal occult blood testing and sigmoidoscopy. Case finding is determined by whether patients are average risk (i.e., over age 40 years) or high-risk (i.e., familial polyposis or Gardner's syndrome, familial colon cancer, female genital cancer, previous adenomas, previous colorectal cancer, and long standing ulcerative colitis). We concentrate here on the screening the high-risk patient group.

### *Familial Polyposis and HNPCC Screening*

Beginning at puberty, patients with a family history of familial polyposis, or Gardner's syndrome, should undergo flexible sigmoidoscopy at least annually. Women with a history of breast or genital cancer in the context of a history of HNPCC, Familial Polyposis syndromes as well as variants, should have yearly fecal occult blood testing and sigmoidoscopy every three years following diagnosis. Patients with FAP and nonpolyposis colorectal carcinoma must be examined colonoscopically beginning at age 20 to 25, or at an age 10 years younger than the index relative. Fecal occult blood testing is not reliable in this very high risk patient population. A reasonable follow-up approach would be annual fecal occult blood testing and three to five yearly colonoscopy.

***Family History of Colorectal Cancer***

There is insufficient evidence supporting the use of colonoscopy as the first step in screening persons with one first-degree relative with colorectal cancer [132]. FOBT and periodic flexible sigmoidoscopy appears more appropriate in this group. More data is needed in groups with two affected first-degree relatives [133]. However, initial colonoscopy at age 40 or at 10 years younger than age of diagnosis of first degree relative, should be followed by routine screening with FOBT and periodic flexible sigmoidoscopy.

***Prior Adenoma or Colorectal Cancer***

Patients in whom colorectal adenoma has been completely excised are likely to develop metachronous neoplasms [134,135]. However, the frequency and time course of future transformations are poorly understood. Approximately one third of patients will develop recurrent adenomas following polypectomy [136]. Some of these early "recurrences" represent missed synchronous adenomas [137]. The presence of multiple adenomas is an important predictor of subsequent adenoma and carcinoma recurrences [138,139]. Other factors that indicate increased risk of recurrence include polyps greater than 1 cm, severe dysplasia, villous structure and older age.

There is uncertainty on the relative importance of each of these factors independently and results of studies are contradictory. Controversy exists over the need for repeated follow-up colonoscopy in patients who have single small adenomas removed [140,141]. Patients with a history of colon cancer resection, should have colonoscopy performed at six months to one year following surgery, followed by a yearly colonoscopy on two occasions. Negative results call for colonoscopy every three years in combination with yearly fecal occult blood testing. Post-operative serum carcinoembryonic antigen (CEA) levels are cost effective for detecting cancer recurrence [142]. Serum CEA levels should be measured at regular intervals, at least three times at four to six-month intervals, then five times at yearly intervals.

## MANAGEMENT

Malignant polyps that invade beyond the muscularis mucosa into the submucosa have metastatic potential, unlike carcinoma *in situ,* which does not invade these layers. Correct diagnosis will influence both management and prognosis, which is also highly dependent on close communication between the endoscopist, surgeon, and pathologist [143]. The ultimate plan of therapy must be individualized according to each patient's medical condition.

## Medical Treatment

Small adenomatous polyps can be reversible lesions. Various trials have been reported with a modest effect on polyp regression following therapy with supplemental fiber, ascorbic acid, and vitamin E in patients with FAP [144]. Sulindac has been shown to decrease the size and number of colorectal adenomas in patients with FAP [145].

However, maintenance on sulindac is not protective against development of rectal cancer, and does not appear to prevent the development of adenomas in children who are genetically susceptible [146].

### *Endoscopic Resection*

Complete endoscopic removal can be curative in adenomas with noninvasive carcinoma, pedunculated adenomas with well-differentiated or moderately differentiated invasive carcinoma, and uncomplicated polypoid carcinomas.

Although most of these lesions are adequately treated by endoscopic polypectomy, about ten percent of patients will have a poor outcome [147] either at the time of polypectomy or on future follow-up. Histopathological features with unfavorable outcomes include poorly differentiated carcinoma, invasion of veins or lymphatics, unclear margins, or $< 2$ mm polypectomy margin, and invasion of bowel wall submucosa. The chance of adverse outcome rises to about 10 to 25 percent in the presence of one or more of these unfavorable features [148].

### *Resectional Surgery*

Total proctocolectomy is the optimal treatment for colonic adenomas, as rectal mucosa that is left behind, is at risk for developing carcinoma. Surgical resection is indicated for malignant polyps in which the invasive carcinoma is poorly differentiated, when it involves endothelium-lined channels (lymphatics, blood vessels), extends to or within 2 mm of the polypectomy margin, or involves the submucosa of the colonic wall including all sessile adenomas.

Total proctocolectomy can be either with a conventional ileostomy or as restorative proctocolectomy with an ileal pouch-anal anastomosis. There are some preferences to subtotal colectomy and ileoproctostomy, but approximately one quarter of patients treated this way subsequently required a total proctectomy for cancer or intractable benign polyps [149]. There have also been reports of spontaneous regression of small rectal polyps in the rectum after surgery.

Consideration of surgical resection should heavily take into account the operative risk, especially in the elderly patient population with comorbid illnesses [150]. For most patients with malignant polyps, polypectomy without surgical resection seems sufficient; however, postpolypectomy endoscopic surveillance should be incorporated into the patients care. Rectal cancers are a significant concern after colectomy, especially in younger patients. In fact, prognosis is quite poor in patients that develop rectal cancer and this has led groups to advocate for total proctocolectomy versus the ileorectal anastomosis, which is preferred by patients for practical purposes. Regardless of the mixed approach and data in this setting, aggressive surveillance is needed of patients who opt for rectal sparing surgeries.

## References

[1] Santero, Michael; Dennis Lee (2005-03-25). "Colon polyp symptoms, diagnosis and treatment". MedicineNet.com. Retrieved 2007-10-25.

[2] Ahlquist DA: Aggressive polyps in hereditary nonpolyposis colorectal cancer: Targets for screening. *Gastroenterology* 1995; 108:1590-2.

[3] Correa, P. Epidemiology of polyps and cancer. In morson, B. C. (ed.). The pathogenesis of Colorectal Cancer. Philadelphia, W. B. Saunders Co. p. 126, 1978.

[4] Rickert, R. R., Auerkbach, O., Garfinkel, L., Hammond, E. C., and Frasca, J. M. Adenomatous lesions of the large bowel: An autopsy survey. *Cancer* 43:1847, 1979.

[5] Clark, J. C., Collan, Y., Eide, T. J., Esteve, H., Ewen, S., Gibbs, N. M., Jensen, O. M., Koskela, E., MacLennan, R., Simpson, J. G., Stalsberg, H., and Zaridze, D. G. Prevalence of polyps in an autopsy series from areas with varying incidence of large bowel cancer. *Int. J. Cancer* 36:179, 1985.

[6] Eide, T. J., and Stalsberg, H. Polyps of the large intestine in northern Norway. *Cancer* 42:2839, 1978.

[7] Stermmermann, G. N., and Yatani, R. Diverticulosis and polyps of the large intestine: A necropsy study of Hawaii Japanese. *Cancer* 31:1260, 1973.
[8] Sato, E., Ouchi, A., Sasano, N., and Ishidate, T. Polyps and diverticulosis of large bowel in autopsy population of Akita prefecture, compared with Miyagi. *Cancer* 37:1316, 1976.
[9] Williams, A. R., Balasooriya, B. A. W., and Day, D. W. Polyps and cancer of the large bowel: A necropsy study in Liverpool. *Gut* 23:835, 1982.
[10] Johson, D. A., Gurney, M. S., Volpe, R. J., Jones, D. M., Van Ness, M., Chobanian, S. J., Avalos, J. C., Buck, J. L., Kooyaman, G., and Cattau, E. L. Jr. A prospective study of prevalence of colonic neoplasms in asymptomatic patients with an age-related risk. *Am. J. Gastroenterol.* 85:969, 1991.
[11] Correa, P. Epidemiology of polyps and cancer. In Morson, B. C. (ed.). The pathogenesis of Colorectal Cancer. Philadelphia. W. B. Saunders Co. p. 126, 1978.
[12] Zaridze, D. G. Environmental etiology of large bowel cancer. *J. Natl. Cancer Inst.* 70:389, 1983.
[13] Armstrong, B., and Doll, R. Environmental factors and cancer incidence and mortality in different countries, with special reference to dietary practices. *Int. J. Cancer* 15:617, 1975.
[14] International Agency for Research on Cancer, Intestinal Microecology Group. Dietary fibre, transit time, faecal bacteria, steroids and colon cancer in two scandinavian populations. *Lancet* 2:207, 1977.
[15] Bingham, S., Williams, D. R., Dole, T. S., and James, W. P. Dietary fiber and regional large bowel mortality in Britain. *Br. J. Cancer* 40: 456, 1979.
[16] Kritchevsky, D. Diet, nutrition and cancer. The role of fiber. Cancer 58:1830, 1986.
[17] Pollack, E. S., Nomura, A. M. Y., Heilbrun, L. K., Stemmermann, G. N., and Green, S. B. Prospective study of alcohol consumption and cancer. *N. Engl. J. Med.* 310:617, 1984.
[18] Kune, S., Kune, G. A., and Watson, L. F. Case-control study of alcoholic beverages as etiological factors: The Melbourne Colorectal Cancer Study. *Nutr. Cancer* 9:43, 1987.
[19] Riboli, E., Cornee, J., Macquart-Moulin, G., Kaaks, R., Casagrande, C., and Guyader, M. Cancer and polyps of the colorectum and lifetime consumption of beer and other alcoholic beverages. *Am. J. Epidemiol.* 133:157, 1991.

[20] Giovannucci, E., Stampfer, M. J., Colditz, G., Rimm, E. B., and Willett, W. C. Relationship of diet to risk of colorectal adenoma in men. *J. Natl. Cancer. Inst.* 84:91, 1992.
[21] Lieberman DA, Prindiville S, Weiss DG, et al: Risk factors for advanced colonic neoplasia and hyperplastic polyps in asymptomatic individuals. *JAMA* 2003; 290:2959-67.
[22] Brahme, F., Ekelund, G., Norden, J. G., and Wenkert, A. Metachronous colorectal polyps. Comparison of development of colorectal polyps and carcinomas in persons with and without histories of polyps. *Dis. Colon. Rectum.* 117:166, 1974.
[23] Bussey, H. J. R. Multiple adenomas and carcinomas. In Morson, B. C (ed.). The pathogenesis of Colorectal Cancer. Philadelphia, W. B. Saunders Co., 1978, p. 72.
[24] Muto, T., Bussey, H. T. R., and Morson, B. C. The evolution of cancer of the colon and rectum. *Cancer* 36:2251, 1975.
[25] Shinya, H., and Wolff, W. I. Morphology, anatomic distribution and cancer potential of colonic polyps. An analysis of 7,000 polyps endoscopically removed. *Ann. Surg.* 190:679, 1979.
[26] Cronkhite, L. W., and Canada, W. J. Generalized gastrointestinal polyposis: an unusual syndrome of polyposis, pigmentation, alopeica nad onychotrophia. *N. Engl. J. Med.* 252:1011, 1955.
[27] O'Briani, D. S., Kennedy, M. J., Daly, P. A., O'Brien, A. A. J., Tanner, W. A., Rogers, P., and Lowlor, E. Multiple lymphomatous polyposis of the gastrointestinal tract. *Am. J. Surg. Pathol.* 13: 691, 1989.
[28] Leppert, M., Dobbs, M., Scambler, P., O'Connell, P., Nakamura, Y., Stauffer, D., Woodward, S., Burt, R., Hughes, J., Gardner, E., Lathrop, M., Wasmuth, J., Lalouel, J. M., and White, R. The gene for familial polyposis coli maps to the long arm of chromosome 5. *Science* 238:1411, 1987.
[29] Solomon, E., Voss, R., Hall, V., Bodmer, W. F., Jass, J. R., Jeffreys, A. J., Lucibello, F. C., Patel I., and RIder, S. H. Chromosome 5 allele loss in human colorectal carcinomas. *Nature* 328:616, 1987.
[30] Groden, J. Thliveris, A., Samowitz, W., Carlson, M., Gelbert, L., Albertsen, H., Joslyn, G., Stevens, J., Spiro, L., Robertson, M., Sargeant, L., Krapcho, K., Wolff, E., Burt, R., Hughes, J. P., Warrington, J., McPherson, J., Wasmuth, J., Le Paslier, D., Abderrahim, H., Cohen, D., Leppert, M., and White, R. Identification and characterization of the familial adenomatous polyposis coli gene. *Cell* 66:589, 1991.

[31] Bussey, H. J. R. Familial Polyposis Coli. Baltimore, Johns Hokins Press, 1975.

[32] Joslyn, G., Carlson, M., Thliveris, A., Albertsen, H., Gelbert, L., Samowitz, W., Groden, J., Stevens, J., Spirio, L., Robertson, M., Sargeant, L., Krapch, K., Wolff, E., Burt, R., Hughes, J. P., Warrington, J., MacPherson, J., Wasmuth, J., LePaslier, D., Abderrahim, H., Cohen, D., Leppert, M., and White, R. Identification of deletion mutations and three new genes at the familial polyposis locus. *Cell* 66:601, 1991.

[33] Nagase, H., Miyoshi, Y., Horii, A., Aoki, T., Ogawa, M., Utsunomiya, J., Baba, S., Sasazuki, T., and Nakamura, Y. Correlation between the location fo germ-line mutations in the APC gene and the number of colocrectal polyps in familial adenomatous polyposis patients. *Cancer* Res. 52:4055, 1992.

[34] Solomon E, Voss R, Hall V, et al: Chromosome 5 allele loss in human colorectal carcinomas. *Nature* 1987; 328:616-19.

[35] Leppert M, Burt R, Hughes JP, Samowitz W, Nakamura Y, Woodward S, et al. Genetic analysis of an inherited predisposition to colon cancer in a family with a variable number of adenomatous polyps. *N. Engl. J. Med.* 1990;322:904–8.

[36] Bussey, H. J. R. Familial Polyposis Coli. Baltimore, Johns Hopkins Press, 1975.

[37] Petersen, G. M., Slack, J., and Nakamura, Y. Screening guidelines and premorbid diagnosis of familial adenomatous polyposis using linkage. *Gastroenterology* 100:1658, 1991.

[38] Bussey HJR: Familial polyposis coli. Baltimore, Johns Hopkins Press, 1975.

[39] Dunlop, M. G., Wyllie, A. H., Steel, C.M., Piris, J, and Evans, H. J. Linked DNA markers for presymptomatic diagnosis of familial adenomatous polyposis. *Lancet* 337:313, 1991.

[40] Utsunomiya, J., and Nakamura, T. The occult osteomatous changes in patients with familial polyposis coli. *Br. J. Surg*. 62:45, 1975.

[41] Jarvinen, H., Nyberg, M., and Peltokallio, P. Upper gastrointestinal tract polyps in familial adenomatous coli. *Gut* 24:333, 1983.

[42] Alexander, J. R., Andrews, J. M., Buchi, K. N., Lee, R. G., Becker, J. M., and Burt, R. W. High prevalence of adenomatous polyps of the duodenal papilla in familial adenomatous polyposis. *Dig. Dis. Sci*. 34:167, 1989.

[43] Tonelli, F., Nardi, F., Bechi, P., Taddei, G., Gozzo, P., and Romagnoli, P. Extracolonic polyps in familial polyposis coli and Gardner's syndrome. *Dis. Colon. Rectum.* 28:664, 1985.

[44] Offerhaus, G. J. A., Giardiello, F. M., Krush, A. J., Booker, S. V., Tersmette, A. C., Kelley, N. C., and Hamilton, S. R. The risk of upper gastrointestinal cancer in familial adenomatous polyposis. *Gastroenterology* 102: 1980, 1992.

[45] Durno C, Monga N, Bapat B, et al: Does early colectomy increase desmoid risk in familial adenomatous polyposis?. *Clin. Gastroenterol. Hepatol.* 2007; 5:1190-4.

[46] Kiel KD, Suit HD: Radiation therapy in the treatment of aggressive fibromatoses (desmoid tumors). *Cancer* 1984; 54:2051-5.

[47] Vasen HF, Möslein G, Alonso A, et al: Guidelines for the clinical management of familial adenomatous polyposis (FAP). *Gut* 2008; 57:704-13.

[48] Tsukada K, Church JM, Jagelman DG, et al: Systemic cytotoxic chemotherapy and radiation therapy for desmoid in familial adenomatous polyposis. *Dis. Colon.*

[49] Stevenson, J. K., and Reid, B. J. Unfamiliar adenomatous polyposis coli. *Am. J. Surg.* 152:81, 1986.

[50] Bussey, H. J. R. Extracolonic lesions associated with polyposis coli. *Proc. R. Med.* 65:294, 1972.

[51] Stevenson, J. K., and Reid, B. J. Unfamiliar adenomatous polyposis coli. *Am. J. Surg.* 152:81, 1986.

[52] Burt, R. W., Riffers, L. F., Gardner, E. J., Lee, R. G., and Tolman, K. G. Villous adenoma of the duodenal papilla presenting as necrotizing pancreatitis in a patient with Gardner's syndrome. *Gastroenterology* 92:523, 1987.

[53] Watanabe, H., Enjoji, M., Yao, T., and Ohsato, K. Gastric lesions in familial adenomatosis coli. *Hum. Pathol.* 9:269, 1978.

[54] Offerhaus, G. J. A., Giardiello, F. M., Krush, A. J., Booker, S. V., Tersmette, A. C., Kelley, N. C., and Hamilton, S. R. The risk of upper gastrointestinal cancer in familial adenomatous polyposis. *Gastroenterology* 102:1980, 1992.

[55] Stevenson, J. K., and Reid, B. J. Unfamiliar aspects of famililа polyposis coli. *Am. Surg.* 152:81, 1986.

[56] Walsh, N., Qizilbash, A., Banerjee, R., and Waugh, G. A. Biliary neoplasia in Gardner's syndrome. *Arch. Pathol. Lab. Med.* 111:76, 1987.

[57] LeSher, A. R., Castronuovo, J. J. Jr., and Filippone, A. L. Jr. Familial polyposis coli and hepatocellular neoplasms. *Surgery* 105:668, 1989.

[58] Garber, J. E., Li, F. P., Kingston, J. E., Krush, A. J., Strong, L. C., Finegold, M. J., Bertario, L., Bulow, S., Filippone, A. Jr., Dedde-Dahl, T. Jr., and Jarvinen, H. J. Hepatoblastoma and familial adenomatous polyposis. *J. Natl. Cancer Inst.* 80: 1616, 1988.

[59] Painter, T. A., and Jagelman, D. G. Adrenal adenomas and adrenal carcinomas in association with hereditary adenomatosis of the colon and rectum. *Cancer* 55:2001, 1985.

[60] Plail, R. O., Bussey, H. J. R., Glazer, G., and Thomson, J. P. S. Adenomatous polyposis: an association with carcinoma of the thyroid. *Br. J. Surg.* 7:377, 1987.

[61] Jones, I. T., Jagelman, D. G., Fazio, V. W., Lavery, I. C., Weakley, F. L., and McGannon, E. Desmoid tumors in familial polyposis coli. *Ann. Surg.* 204:94, 1986.

[62] Klemmer, S., Pascoe, L., and DeCosse, J. Occurence of desmoid tumors in patients with famlial adenomatous polyposis of the colon. *Am. J. Med. Genet.* 28:385, 1987.

[63] Burn J, Chapman P, Delhanty J, et al: The UK northern region genetic register for familial adenomatous polyposis coli: use of age of onset, congenital hypertrophy of the retinal pigment epithelium, and DNA markers in risk calculations. *J. Med. Genet.* 1991; 28:289-96.

[64] Blair NP, Trempe CL: Hypertrophy of the retinal pigment epithelium associated with Gardner's syndrome. *Am. J. Ophthalmol.* 1980; 90:661-7.

[65] Turcot, J., Despres, J. P., and St. Pierre, T. Malignant tumors of the central nervous system associated with familial polyposis of the colon. Report of two cases. *Dis. Colon. Rectum.* 2:465, 1959.

[66] Jarvis, L., Bathurst, N., Mohan, D., and Beckly, D. Turcot's syndrome - a review. *Dis. Colon. Rectum.* 31:907, 1988.

[67] Costa, O. L., Silva, D. M., Colnago, R. A., Vieira, M. S., and Musso, C. Turcot syndrome - autosomal dominant or recessive transmission? *Dis. Colon. Rectum.* 30:391, 1987.

[68] Itoh, H., and Ohsato, K. Turcot syndrome and its characteristic colonic manifestations. *Dis. Colon. Rectum.* 28:399, 1985.

[69] Boland, C. R. Familial colonic cancer syndromes. West. *J. Med.* 138:351, 1983.

[70] Anderson, D. E. An inherited form of large bowel cancer. Muir's sundrome. *Cancer* 45:103, 1980.

[71] Rutgerts, P., Hendricks, H., Geboes, K., Ponette, E., Broeckaert, L., and Vantrappen, G. Involvement of the upper digestive tract by systemic neurofibromatosis. *Gastrointest. Endosc.* 27:22, 1981.

[72] Cowden's syndrome,(Salem, O. S., and Steck, W. D. Cowden's disease (multiple hamartoma and neoplasia syndrome). *J. Am. Acad. Dermatol.* 8:686, 1983.

[73] Schwartz, R. A. Basal cell nevus syndrome and gastrointestinal polyposis. *N. Engl. J. Med.* 299:49, 1978.

[74] Foley, T. R., McGarrity, T. J., and Abt, A. B. Peutz-Jeghers syndrome: A clinicopathologic survey of the "Harrisburg Family" with a 49-year follow-up. *Gastroenterology* 95:1535, 1988.

[75] Burdick, D., and Prior, J. T. Peutz-Jeghers syndrome. A clinicopathologic study of a large family with a 27-year follow-up. *Cnacer* 50:2139, 1982.

[76] Howell, J., Pringle, K., Kirschner, B., and Burrington, J. D. Peutz-Jeghers polyps causing colocolic intussusception in infancy. *J. Pediatr. Surg.* 16:82, 1981.

[77] Konishi, F., Wyse, N. E., Muto, T., Sawada, T., Morioka, Y., Sugmura, H., and Yamaguchi, K. Peutz-Jeghers polyposis associated with carcinoma of the digestive organs. *Dis. Colon. Rectum.* 30:790, 1987.

[78] Miller, L. J., Bartholomew, L. G., Dozois, R. R., and Dahlin, D. C. Adenoccarcinoma of the rectum arising in a hamartomatous polyhp in a pateint with Peutz-Jeghers syndrome. *Dig. Dis. Sci.* 28:1047, 1983.

[79] Scully, R. E. Sex cord tumor with annular tubules. A distinctive ovarian tumor of the Peutz-Jeghers syndrome. *Cancer* 25:1107, 1970.

[80] Wilson, D. M., Pitts, W. C., Hintz, R. I., and Rosenfeld, R. G. Testicular umors with Peutz-Jeghers syndrome. *Cancer* 57:2238, 1986.

[81] Bowlby, L. S. Pancereatic adenocarcinoma in an adolescent male with peutz-Jeghers syndrome. *Hum. Pathol.* 17:97, 1986.

[82] Wada, K., Tanaka, M., Yamaguchi, K., and Wada, K. Carcinoma and polyps of the gallbladder associated with Peutz-Jeghers syndrome. *Dig. Dis. Sci.* 32:943, 1987.

[83] Giardiello FM, Brensinger JD, Tersmette AC, et al: Very high risk of cancer in familial Peutz-Jeghers syndrome. *Gastroenterology* 2000; 119:1447-53.

[84] Calva D, Howe JR: Hamartomatous polyposis syndromes. *Surg. Clin. North Am.* 2008; 88:779-817.

[85] Stemper, T. J., Kent, T. H., and Summers, R. W. Juvenile polyposis and gastrointestinal carcinoma. A study of a kindred. *Ann. Intern. Med.* 83:639, 1975.

[86] Bresalier, R. S., and Toribara, N. W. Familial colon cancer. In Eastwood, G. L. (ed.). Premalignant Conditions of the Gastrointestinal Tract. Controversies in Gastoenterology Series. D. Zakim (ed.). New York, Elsevier Science Publishers, 1990, p. 227.

[87] Markowitz, J. F., Aiges, H. W., Cunningham-Rundles, S., Kahn, E., Teichbert, S., Fisher, S. E., and Daum, F. Cancer family syndrome: Marker studies. *Gastroenterology* 91:581, 1986.

[88] Lynch, H. T., Kimberling, W., Albano, W. A., Lynch, S, F., Biscone, K., Schuelke, G., S, Sandberg, A. A., Lipkin, M., Deschner, E. E., Mikol, Y. B., Elston, R. C., Bailey-Wilson, J. E., and Danes, B. S. Hereidtary nonpolyposis colorectal cancer (Lynch syndrome I and II). II. Biomarker studies. *Cancer* 56:939, 1985.

[89] Lanspa, S. J., Lynch, H. T., Smyrk, T. C., Strayhorn, P., Watson, P., Lynch, J. F., Jenkins, J. X., and Appleman, H. D. Colorecatl adenomas in the Lynch syndromes. Results of a colonoscopy screeing program. *Gastroenterology* 98:1117, 1990.

[90] Mecklin, J. P., Sipponen. P., and Jarvinen, J. H. Histopathology of colorectal carcinomas and adenomas in cancer family syndrome. *Dis. Colon. Rectum.* 29:849, 1986.

[91] Klein, I., Parveen, G., Gavaler, J. S., and Van Thiel, D. H. Colonic polyps in patients with acromegaly. *Ann. Intern. Med.* 97:27, 1982.

[92] Pines, A., Rozen, P., Ron, E., and Gilat. T. Gastrointestinal tumors in acromegalic patients. *Am. J. Gastroenterol.* 80:266, 1985.

[93] Brunner, J. E., Johnson, C. C., Zafar, S., Peterson, E. L., Brunner, J. F., and Mellinger, R. C. Colon cancer and polyps in acromegaly: Increased risk associated with family history of colon cancer. *Clin. Endocrinol.* 32:65, 1990.

[94] Brunner, J. E., Johnson, C. C., Zafar, S., Peterson, E. L., Brunner, J. F., and Mellinger, R. C. Colon cancer and polyps in acromegaly: Increased risk associated with family history of colon cancer. *Clin. Endocrinol.* 32:65, 1990.

[95] Ezzat, S., Strom, C., Melmed, S. Colon polyps in acromegaly. *Ann. Intern. Med.* 114:754, 1991.

[96] Cats A, Dullaart RP, Kleibeuker JH, et al: Increased epithelial cell proliferation in the colon of patients with acromegaly. *Cancer Res.* 1996; 56:523-6.

[97] Jenkins PJ, Frajese V, Jones AM, et al: Insulin-like growth factor I and the development of colorectal neoplasia in acromegaly. *J. Clin. Endocrinol.*

[98] Klein, R. S., Catalano, M. T., Edberg, S. C., Casey, J. I., and Steigbigel, N . H. Streptococcus bovis septicemia and carcinoma of the colon. *Ann. Intern. Med.* 9:560, 1979.

[99] Marshall, J. B., and Gerhardt, D. C. Polyposis coli presenting with Streptococcus bovis endocarditis. *Am. J. Gastroenterol.* 75:314, 1981.

[100] Klein, R. S., Recco, R. A., Catalano, M. T., Edberg, S. C., Casey, J. I., and Steigbigel, N. H. Association of Streptococcus bovis with carcinoma of the colon. *N. Engl. J. Med.* 297:800, 1977.

[101] Stewart, M., Macrae, F. A., and Williams, C. B. Neoplasia and ureterosigmoidostomy: A colonoscopic survey. *Br. J. Surg.* 69:414, 1982.

[102] Ali, M. H., Satti, M. B., and Al-nafussi, A. Multiple benign colonic polyps at the site of ureterosigmoidostomy. *Cancer* 53: 1006, 1984.

[103] Stewart, M., Hill, M. J., Pugh, R. C. B., and Williams, J. P. The role of N-nitrosamine in carcinogenesis at the ureterocolic anastomosis. *Br. J. Urol.* 53:115, 1981.

[104] Correa, P, Strong, J. P., Johnson, W. D., Pizzolato, P., and Haenszel, W. Atherosclerosis and polyps of the colon. Quantification of precursors of coronary heart disease and colon cancer. *J. Chronic Dis.* 35: 313, 1982.

[105] Stemmermann, G. N., Heilbrun, L. K., Nomra, A., Yano, K., and Hayashi, T. Adenomatous polyps and atherosclerosis: An autopsy study of Japanese men in Hawaii. *Int. J. Cancer* 38:789, 1986.

[106] Winawer, S. J., Flehinger, B. J., Buchalter, J., Herbert, E., and Shike, M. Declining serum cholesterol levels prior to diagnosis of colon cancer. *J.A.M.A.* 263:2083, 1990.

[107] Neugut, A. I., Murray, T. I., Garbowski, G. C., Forde, K. A., Treat, M. R., Waye, J. D., and Fenoglio-Preiser, C. Cholecystectomy as a risk factor for colorectal adenomatous polyps and carcinoma. *Cancer* 68:1644, 1991.

[108] Bandettini, L., Filipponi, F., and Romagnoli, P. Increase of the mitotic index of colonic mucosa after cholecystectomy. *Cancer* 58:685, 1986.

[109] Sobin, L. H. The histopathology of bleeding from polyps and carcinomas of the large intestine. *Cancer* 55:577, 1985.
[110] Waldock, A., Ellis, I. O., and Armitage, N. C. M. Histopathological assessment of bleeding from polyps of the colon and rectum. *J. Clin. Pathol.* 42:378, 1989.
[111] Shnitka, T. K., Friedman, M. H. W., Kidd, E. G., and MacKenzie, W. C. Villous tumors of the rectum and colon characterized by severe fluid and electrolyte loss. *Surg. Gynecol. Obstet.* 112: 609, 1961.
[112] Duthie, H. L., and Atwell, J. D. The absorption of water, sodium, and potassium in the large intestine with particular reference to the effects of villous papillomas. *Gut* 4:373, 1963.
[113] Silman, A. J., Mitchell, P. Nicholls, R. J., Macrea, F. A., Leicester, R. J., Bartram, C. I., Simmons, M. J., Campbell, P. D. J., Hearn, C. E. D., and Constable, P. J. Self-reported dark red bleeding as a marker comparable with occult blood testing in screeing for large bowel neoplasms. *Br. J. Surg*. 70:721, 1983.
[114] Guillem, J. G., Forde, K. A., Treat, M. R., Neugut, A. I., and Bodian, C. A The impact of colonoscopy on the early detection of colonic neoplasms in patients with rectal bleeding. *Ann. Surg.* 206:606, 1987.
[115] Macrae, F., and St. John, D. J. B. Relationship between patterns of bleeding and Hemoccult sensitivity in patients with colorectal cancers of adenomas. *Gastroenterology* 82:891, 1982.
[116] Herzog, P., Holtermuller, K., Preiss, J., Fischer, J., Ewe, K., Schreiber, H., and Berres, M. Fecal blood loss chromium labeled erythrocytes and with the Hemoccult test. *Gastroenterology* 83:957, 1982.
[117] Gabrielsson, N., Granqvist, S., and Nilsson, B. Guaiac tests detection of occult faecal blood loss in patients with endoscopically verified colonic polyps. *Scand. J. Gastroenterol*. 20:978, 1985.
[118] Norfleet, R. G. Effect of diet on fecal occult blood testing in patients with colorectal polyps. *Dig. Dis. Sci*. 31:498, 1986.
[119] Marks, G., Boggs, H. W., Castro, A. F., Gathright, J. B., Ray, J. E., and Salvati, E. Sigmoidoscopic examinations with rigid and flexible fiberoptic sigmoidoscopes in the surgeon's office: A comparative prospective study of effectiveness in 1,012 cases. *Dis. Colon. Rectum*. 22:162, 1979.
[120] Bohlman, T. W., Katon, R. M., Lipschutz, G. R., McCool, M. F., Smith, F. W., and Melnyk, C. S. Fiberoptic pansigmoidoscopy: An evaluation and comparison with rigid sigmoidoscopy. *Gastroenterology* 72:644, 1977.

[121] Winnan, G., Berci, G., Panish, J., Talbot, T. M., Overholt, B. F., and McCallum, R. W. Superiority of the flexible to the rigid sigmoidoscope in routine proctosigmoidoscopy. *N. Engl. J. Med.* 302:1011, 1980.

[122] McCallum, R. W., Meyer, C. T., Marignani, P., Cane, E., and Contino, C. Flexible sigmoidoscopy: Diagnostic yield in 1015 patients. *Am. J. Gastroenterol.* 79:433, 1984.

[123] Zucker, G. M., Madura, M. J., Chmiel, J. S., and Olinger, E. J. The advantage of the 30-cm flexible sigmoidoscope over the 60-cm flexible sigmoidoscope. *Gastrointest. Endosc.* 30:59, 1984.

[124] Sarles, H. E., Jr., Sanowski, R. A., Haynes, W. C., and Bellapravus, S. The long and short of flexible sigmoidoscopy: Does it matter? *Am. J. Gastroenterol.* 81:369, 1986.

[125] Ott, D. J., Chen, Y. M., Gelfand, D. W., Wu, W. C., and Munitz, H. A. Single-contrast vs double-contrast barium enema in the detection of colonic polyps. *A. J. R.* 146: 933, 1986.

[126] Williams, C. B., Hunt, R. H., Loose, H., Riddell, R. H., Sakai, Y., and Swarbrick, E. T. Colonoscopy in the management of colon polyps. *Br. J. Surg.* 61: 673, 1974.

[127] Williams, C. B., Macrae, F. A., and Bartrum, C. I. A prospective study of diagnostic methods in adenoma follow-up. *Endoscopy* 14:74, 1982.

[128] Thoeni, R. F., and Menuck, L. Comparison of barium enema and colonoscopy in the detection of samll colonic polyps. *Radiology* 124: 631, 1977.

[129] Swarbrick, E. T., Fevre, D. I. , Hunt, R. H., Thomas, B. M., and Williams, C. B. Colonoscopy for unexplained rectal bleeding. *Br. J. Med.* 2:1685, 1978.

[130] Aldridge, M. C., and Sim, A. J. W. Colonoscopy findings in symptomatic patients without X-ray evidence of colonic neoplasms. *Lancet* 2:833, 1986.

[131] Mathus-Vliegen, E. M. H., and Tytgat, G. N. J. Nd:YAG laser photocoagulation in colorectal adenoma. *Gastroenterology* 90:1865, 1986.

[132] Rozen, P., Fireman, Z., and Figer, A. Family history of colorectal cancer as a marker of potential malignancy within a screening program. *Cancer* 60:248, 1987.

[133] Grossman, S., and Milos, M. L. Colonoscopic screening of persons with suspected risk factors for colon cancer. I. Family history. *Gastroenterology* 94:395, 1988.

[134] Kune, G. A., Kune, S., and Watson, L. F. History of colorectal polypectomy and risk of subsequent colorectal cancer. *Br. J. Surg.* 74:1064, 1987.

[135] Brahme, F., Ekelund, G. R., Norden, J. G., and Wenkert, A. Metachronous colorectal polyps: Comparison of development of colorectal polyps and carcinomas in persons with and without histories of polyps. *Dis. Colon. Rectum.* 17:166, 1974.

[136] Henry, L. G., Condon, R. E., Schulte, W. J., Aprahamian, C., and DeCosse, J. J. Risk of recurrence of colon polyps. *Ann. Surg.* 182:511, 1975.

[137] Waye, J. D., and Braunfeld, S. Surveillance intervals after colonoscopic polypectomy. *Endoscopy* 14:79, 1981.

[138] Williams, C. B. The logic and logistics of colon polyp follow-up. In Glass, G. B. J., and Sherlock, P. (eds.). Progress in Gastroenterology. vol. 4. New York, Grune and Stratton, p. 513, 1983.

[139] Matek, W., Guggenmoos-Holzmann, I., and Demling, L. Follow-up of patients with colorectal adenomas. *Endoscopy* 17:175, 1985.

[140] Grossman, S., Milos, M. L., Tekawa, I. S., and Jewell, N. P. Colonoscopic screening of persons with suspected risk factors for colon cancer. II. Past history of colorectal neoplasms. *Gastroeneterology* 96:299, 1989.

[141] Achkar, E., and Carey, W. Small polyps found during fiberoptic sigmoidoscopy in asymptomatic patients. *Ann. Intern. Med.* 109:880, 1988.

[142] Deveny, K. E., and Way, L. W. Follow-up of patients with colorectal cancer. *Am. J. Surg.* 148:717, 1984.

[143] Haggitt, R. C., Glotzbach, R. E., Soffer, E. E., and Wruble, L. D. Prognostic factors in colorectal acrcinoma arising in adenomas: Implications for lesions removed by endoscopic polypectomy. Gastroenterology 89:328, 1985. (Riddell, R. H. Hands off "cancerous" large bowel polyps. *Gastroenterology* 89:432, 1985.

[144] DeCosse JJ, Miller HH, Lesser ML: Effect of wheat fiber and vitamins C and E on rectal polyps in patients with familial adenomatous polyposis. *J. Natl. Cancer Inst.* 1989; 81:1290-7.

[145] Levin TR, Palitz A, Grossman S, et al: Predicting advanced proximal colonic neoplasia with screening sigmoidoscopy. *JAMA* 1999; 281:1611-17.

[146] Giardiello FM, Yang VW, Hylind LM, et al: Primary chemoprevention of familial adenomatous polyposis with sulindac. *N. Engl. J. Med.* 2002; 346:1054-9.

[147] Wilcox, G. M., Anderson, P. B., and Colacchio, T. A. Early invasive carcinoma in colonic polyps: A review of the literature

with emphasis on the assessment of the risk of metastasis. *Cancer* 57:160, 1986.

[148] Nugent KP, Talbot IC, Hodgson SV, et al: Solitary juvenile polyps: not a marker for subsequent malignancy. *Gastroenterology* 1993; 105:698-700.

[149] Skinner MA, Tyler D, Branum GE, et al: Subtotal colectomy for familial polyposis. *Arch. Surg.* 1990; 125:621-4.

[150] Wilcox, G. M., and Beck, J. R. Early invasive cancer in adenomatous colonic polyps ("malignant polyps"): Evaluation of the therapeutic options by dedision analysis. *Gastroenterology* 92:1159, 1987.

In: Dysplasia
Editors: L. M. Sexton and H. J. Leach
ISBN 978-1-61942-600-9


*Chapter II*

# Developmental Dysplasia of Hip

***Bilal Jamal and Anand Pillai***
MRCS - Specialty Registrar, Trauma and Orthopaedics,
West of Scotland rotation, UK
FRCS - Consultant Orthopaedic Surgeon,
Ninewell's Hospital, Dundee

## Abstract

Developmental dysplasia of hip presents with a spectrum of disease. The natural history of it is poorly appreciated and for this reason, the exact role of various screening programmes and treatments is also poorly understood. Correspondingly, different nations have pursued differing strategies for treating infants with developmental dysplasia of hip.

In this chapter, we review the terminology to be aware of, the risk factors and various presentations of hip dysplasia as well as the importance of clinical examination and the role of imaging studies.

Screening is controversial and we rehearse the arguments for and against it. We also discuss the various treatments options available; these are dependent upon the age of presentation.

## INTRODUCTION

Developmental Dysplasia of Hip (DDH) is a term that encompasses a spectrum of disease. It refers to abnormalities of the femoral head, the acetabulum or, indeed, both. The unstable hip may well be dysplastic, subluxed, dislocatable or dislocatable and irreducible. A dysplastic hip is one in which the hip joint is concentric but can be provoked to sublux. A subluxed hip arises when the femoral head only partially articulates with the acetabulum while in frank dislocation, there is no articulation between the head and acetabulum.

The irreducible dislocation is commonly known as a teratological dislocation. This is a distinct form of DDH in which the hip joint is dislocated prior to birth, there is a limited range of motion and the hip is irreducible on examination. It tends to be associated with other childhood conditions such as myelopdysplasia, Larsen's syndrome, multiple epiphyseal dysplasia and Trevor's disease [1]. Amongst those with cerebral palsy, 35% will be troubled by DDH [2].

In 1989, Klisic [3] introduced the term DDH after recognising that the previous diagnostic label of congenital dislocation of hip was inaccurate. Not all hips are dislocated at birth but may go onto become dysplastic with age. Accordingly, there has been a move away from referring to late diagnosed cases of DDH as "missed." They are now referred to as "late" cases in an attempt to acknowledge that the hip may have been normal upon clinical examination at birth but has since become dysplastic.

## HIP DEVELOPMENT

An understanding of normal and pathological hip development is vital if one is to appreciate the rationale that underpins the various treatments available. The hip joint begins to develop at the seventh week of gestation when a cleft appears within the mesenchyme of the limb bud. By the eleventh week of gestation, a cartilaginous hip joint complex is formed. At birth, the acetabulum is composed of cartilage with a fibrocartilaginous rim known as labrum. The acetabular cartilage is continuous with the triradiate cartilage. The proximal femur is entirely cartilaginous in nature at birth. Between the fourth and seventh post natal months, the proximal femoral ossification centre appears. Growth of the proximal femur is affected by numerous factors including muscle pull, joint nutrition, muscle tone and forces transmitted across the joint.

A tight fit is possible between the femoral head and acetabulum in normality. This is, in part, due to the surface tension created by synovial fluid. In those with DDH, the femoral head can sublux out of joint as this tight fit is not possible. The possible pathological changes that can be found at birth are varied. However, the most common is that of a hypertrophied ridge of acetabular cartilage along the superior, posterior and inferior aspects of the acetabulum. This is commonly referred to as the "neolimbus" and it is over this structure that the femoral head subluxes out of the acetabulum producing a characteristic palpable sign.

In those hips that remain chronically dislocated, secondary restraints to closed reduction can develop. Fatty tissue, known as pulvinar, thickens and impedes reduction. Ligamentum teres can also thicken again blocking reduction. Transverse acetabular ligament becomes hypertrophic and inferior capsule develops a hourglass shape which prevents closed reduction.

## EPIDEMIOLOGY

The incidence of DDH is dependent upon numerous factors. It varies according to the age of the child and the method of clinical assessment. Amongst an unscreened population of principally European descent, clinically diagnosed DDH is found to be in the order of 1.3 per 1000. When clinical screening programmes are employed, using tests such as Ortolani and Barlow manoeuvres, the incidence is increased; it can be as high as 28.5 per 1000 [9]. The incidence of ultrasonagraphically detected DDH is higher yet [10].

Risk factors for DDH are well described and include breech presentation, female sex, family history and firstborn status. Up to a third of those affected by DDH have a positive family history [4, 5]. In the majority of cases, females are affected [6]. This may well be because of increased ligamentous laxity as a result of extra oestrogen produced by the female foetus. DDH is more common amongst those who are born in the breech position [7]. This may well be due to hamstring forces, from an extended knee, acting on the hip joint leading to a dysplastic hip. It is thought that any situation which leads to less intrauterine space for the foetus can lead to DDH. Hence the reason for why oligohydramnios and large birth weight lead to DDH. Racial variation in DDH has been noted such that the incidence of DDH in Chinese and African babies is almost 0% while it is 1% for hip dysplasia in Caucasian babies [8]. These differences could be due to child rearing practices rather than genetic influences. African children are usually carried with the legs in a flexed and abducted position. This is the optimum position for hip stability. Native American children, however, are carried with the hips in extension. This increases tension within psoas which could allow for the hip joint to sublux or dislocate. Other risk factors include torticollis, metatarsus adductus and delivery by caesarean section.

## Clinical Presentation

The clinical presentation of a child with DDH very much varies according to their age. In neonates, DDH is diagnosed by the Ortolani and Barlow tests. It can also be diagnosed by a grossly abnormal ultrasound examination of the hip. Ortolani first described his eponymous test in 1937 [11] while Barlow described his test in 1962 [12].

Ortolani's test attempts to identify the dislocated or subluxed hip which is reducible. It is performed with the child suitably exposed in the supine position. Both hips should be flexed to 90 degrees but each hip should be examined separately. One's index and middle fingers are placed over the child's greater trochanter. The thumb is placed medially near the groin crease. The pelvis is stabilised by holding the contralateral hip still. The hip being examined should be slowly abducted while passing an upward force through the greater trochanter. An abnormal finding is recorded when a "clunk" is palpated. This "clunk" represents the relocation of a dislocated femoral head into the acetabulum.

Barlow's test aims to identify the dislocatable hip. It is performed by positioning the patient as for Ortolani's test. The contralateral hip is again stabilised. The hip is adducted and a gentle downward pressure is exerted in an attempt to sublux the hip posteriorly. It is useful to note that both these tests are helpful in the child who is younger than 3 months. Thereafter, soft tissue restraints limit motion of the hip. Despite the fact that both tests are used commonly in many developed countries routinely, the interobserver agreement is poor and there is poor consensus on what represents an acceptable examination [13, 14].

In the older infant, one of approximately three months, other useful clinical signs can be elicited. Limited abduction as compared to the contralateral hip points towards a diagnosis of DDH [15] and is thought to be due to shortening of the adductor muscles associated with subluxation or dislocation of the hip. The affected thigh may also be noted to be shortened as compared to the contralateral limb; this is referred to as galeazzi's sign. It is most pronounced when the hips are placed in 90 degrees of flexion and the height of the knees is compared. The shortening is thought to be due to hip dislocation or congenital femoral shortening. Asymmetric thigh skin folds are suggestive of DDH but are not a specific sign.

A particular diagnostic challenge clinically presents itself in a child with bilateral DDH. They have limited abduction in both hips and their thighs are of similar length. In such a case, Klisic's test can be useful. One's long finger is placed upon the greater trochanter while the index finger is placed over the anterior superior iliac spine. In normality, a line drawn between the two fingers will point to the umbilicus. In a case of DDH, the line will run distal to the umbilicus. This is because, in the dislocated hip, the trochanter is elevated.

In the previously undiagnosed walking child, there is often a history of limping, waddling gait, tip toe walking or of dragging one leg. Examination reveals an abnormal trendelenburg sign and a trendelenburg gait. Limited abduction of the hip along with an abnormal galeazzi sign will be evident. Exaggerated lumbar lordosis may well also be present as a result of hip flexion contracture.

## IMAGING

The aim of imaging is to confirm a diagnosis of DDH. This is commonly done via ultrasonagraphy. It is important to have an appreciation of physiological ranges of laxity to prevent overtreatment. Ultrasound is also useful at confirming and monitoring hip joint reduction in treatment devices. Radiographs are particularly useful in the infant older than six months as by that point the proximal femoral epiphysis has ossified. In this age of infant, radiographs can confirm a diagnosis of DDH. In the older infant, they also have a role in the pre-operative assessment of those who need corrective ostetomies.

In infants younger than 6 months, the hip joint is cartilaginous in nature and, therefore, ultrasound is the imaging modality of choice. It has been used in the context of screening, to examine those with risk factors for DDH and to further assess those with an abnormal clinical assessment. It also has an important role in assessing response to and length of treatment. Graf is credited with many of the advances in sonagraphy for DDH. He has proposed that ultrasound can assess hip morphology [16]. Graf suggests that each hip can be assigned to one of four categories on the basis of the acetabulum, the bony modelling, and the cartilage roof. In essence, type one hips are considered normal, type two hips are either physiologically immature or moderately abnormal, type three and four consist of eccentric hips with poor bony modelling, flattened bony rims and a displaced cartilage roof triangle. Type one hips require no follow up. Type three and four hips require treatment. The management of type two hips is more controversial. Some authorities would place all patients with a type two hip in an abduction brace whilst others will only do so after taking account of the clinical picture.

Harcke proposes a dynamic method of hip sonagraphy where hip stability and the relationship between the femoral head and acetabulum is emphasised [17]. Each hip is classified as normal, subluxed or dislocated.

The overwhelming advantage of ultrasound is the lack of ionising radiation. However, its high cost, limited availability and lack of trained sonagraphers restrict its use. Ultrasound is also limited by its inadequate sensitivity and specificity. The Norwegian experience points to a sensitivity of 88.5% and a positive predictive value of 61.6% [18]. This may result in overtreatment of patients leading to higher healthcare costs.

Radiographs are of use in the infant who is older than 6 months as it is at this point that the proximal femoral epiphysis ossifies (range two to eight months [19]). An anteroposterior view of the pelvis is useful to assess for DDH. It also has a role in assessing hip development following treatment as well as monitoring for longer term outcomes. In addition to an anteroposterior radiograph, films with the hip in abduction and internal rotation are necessary. These demonstrate whether the hip is reducible.

An awareness of several reference lines is crucial to reproducibly interpret pelvis radiographs in an infant. Hilgenreiner's line is a horizontal line drawn through the triradiate cartilages of the pelvis. Perkin's line is a vertical line that is drawn perpendicularly to Hilgenreiner's line. It is drawn through the most lateral ossified margin of each acetabulum. In normality, the femoral head lies within the inferomedial quadrant of the intersection of the two lines. Shenton's line is drawn along the medial border of the femoral neck and should run in continuity with the inferior border of the superior pubic ramus. This line is disrupted in those with DDH.

An important angle to assess on a pelvic radiograph is that of the acetabular index which is formed by the intersection between Hilgenreiner's line and a line from the inferior aspect of the iliac bone to the most lateral margin of the roof of acetabulum. This value varies with age but by the age of four months, it should be no more than 25 degrees. After fusion of the triradiate cartilage, the centre edge angle of Wiberg is a useful method of assessing lateral coverage of the femoral head. It is defined as the angle between Perkin's line and a line from the lateral most edge of acetabulum to the centre of the femoral head.

## SCREENING

The rationale behind screening for DDH is that earlier diagnosis will lead to simpler treatments resulting in better outcomes and minimising the need for complex surgical treatments that are needed for those who present late. While there is general agreement that screening is needed, there is little agreement upon the method to use. There is a paucity of evidence to inform the debate and controversy regarding the precise form of screening to use looks likely to persist.

There is widespread consensus within developed countries that all neonates should be assessed clinically, via the Ortolani and Barlow tests, for DDH. Beyond this statement, there is little agreement upon what should constitute standard practice for hip screening.

The concern with clinical screening relates to its poor sensitivity even when being performed by an experienced clinician [20]. It may be that because of the poor sensitivity of clinical examination, there are numerous patients who had DDH at birth which was not identified. This is clearly distressing for the families and clinicians involved; it also presents medico-legal difficulties.

In acknowledgement of the above difficulties, some countries, such as Austria and Germany, have moved to a programme of universal sonagraphic assessments of hips. This has not been replicated within other western countries. Universal screening programmes can lead to gross overtreatment of neonates. In one series, 9% of children required hip splintage [21]. In another series, higher rates of abduction splinting were again recorded. The authors noted that in those who were screened with ultrasound, there was a lower rate of late DDH; this was not statistically significant however [18].

Overtreatment is not benign. It leads to significant parental anxiety and raises the possibility of pressure sores as well as femoral nerve palsies. Splinting is associated with a 1% risk of avascular necrosis and ultimately osteoarthritis; this should caution against overtreatment and is one why reason why universal sonagraphic screening has not been more widely adopted. Other practical considerations that have limited its uptake include its expense and the need for trained sonagraphers.

In 2006, the US preventive services task force concluded that there is insufficient evidence to recommend routine screening for DDH in infants as a means to prevent future complications [22].

Selective hip sonagraphy, targeted at those neonates with risk factors for DDH, may well be the answer but the case is yet to be convincingly made.

## Management

The aim of treatment in DDH is to obtain and maintain a reduced, congruent hip joint in order to minimise the likelihood of degenerative joint disease in the longer term. The treatment necessary is very much dependent upon the age at which diagnosis is made. The earlier that treatment is instituted, the simpler it is to perform and the better the long term result is likely to be due to the greater potential for remodelling of both the acetabulum and femur.

Hip instability may be noted clinically at birth. It requires no specific treatment as it can be transient and resolve within the first two weeks of life as joint laxity diminishes. These patients do require to be followed up. If hip instability persists beyond two weeks, it requires treatment. Treatment at two weeks is not associated with poorer outcomes than if treatment were instituted immediately [23].

Historically, infants were placed in double or triple nappies. There is no role for such diapers as it seems they provide false reassurance and are no more effective than placebo. They do, however, have the potential to cause avascular necrosis of the hip.

In DDH, the hip is reduced in abduction and flexion. Therefore, splinting the neonatal hip in this position allows for the maintenance of a concentric reduction of the hip allowing for an improvement in the underlying dysplasia. The position in which the hip is placed is critical. If too much flexion and abduction is applied, the blood supply to the femoral head can be compromised leading to avascular necrosis; this occurs in approximately 1% of patients. A compromise must be made between placing the hip in enough flexion and abduction that it is stable while ensuring it is not such an extreme position that the blood supply is threatened. A safe position to adopt is one of 100 degrees of flexion and thirty to sixty degrees of abduction.

Various forms of splits are available. These can be divided into rigid splints such as the Van Rosen splint which remains widely used in the United Kingdom or dynamic splints such as the Pavlik splint which is the most popular worldwide. Hip spica casts are also available.

Van Rosen splints hold the hips in a fixed position, they have the advantage of being easy to apply but potential complications include the risk of avascular necrosis, pressure sores, loss of reduction as well as injury to the accessory nerve as the splint is attached to the shoulder area.

Pavlik splints have the advantage that they allow for some hip motion; this allows for the acetabulum to be moulded by the femoral head and aims to protect against avascular necrosis. However, it remains possible as does the risk of femoral nerve palsy and loss of reduction. They are contraindicated in those with gross muscle imbalance or ligamentous laxity. Patients are examined clinically and sonagraphically on a weekly basis with hip stability usually being established within the first 3 weeks of treatment. The ideal duration of splintage has not yet been established but one suggestion is that treatment should persist for 6 weeks following establishment of a stable and congruent joint. Treatment is a Pavlik splint is associated with a 95% success rate in dysplasia and subluxation whilst it is only 80% in dislocation. If treatment in a Pavlik harness is instituted after six months of age, the success rate is less than 50%. This is because of the difficulty in maintaining a splint in an increasingly active infant.

If after 3 weeks reduction of the hip is not achieved, splintage should be abandoned. Rather, closed reduction under anaesthesia should be attempted with a hip spica cast being applied thereafter.

Special mention should be made of the tetatogenic or irreducible hip. Splintage should not be employed in these cases as the hip will not be reduced but rather the blood supply will be compromised raising the spectre of avascular necrosis. In these cases, the optimal treatment is to pursue closed reduction from the age of 3 months onwards. At this point, it is sensible to consider an arthrogram, examination under anaesthetic and an adductor tenotomy. If, despite this, a closed reduction is not possible then an open reduction should be considered from the age of four months onwards.

In the child between the ages of six to twenty four months, closed or open reduction of the dislocated hip is necessary. Some authorities precede this by traction for a period of three weeks in an attempt to decrease muscular contracture and thus allow for a gentler closed reduction.

Closed reduction is always performed in theatre under general anaesthesia. A dislocated hip is reduced gently with a mixture of flexion, traction and adduction. After reduction is achieved, it is imperative to assess stability. The hip is moved through a range of motion to determine the range within which it will stay reduced. A "safe zone" can be determined; it is a large area then the reduction is taken to be stable. If, however, the extremes of abduction or internal rotation are required to achieve and maintain reduction then the reduction is taken to be unstable. In this case, an adductor tenotomy is often required. An arthrogram can help is assessing the stability of reduction. After reduction, a hip spica cast is applied to maintain reduction and a radiograph taken to confirm maintenance of reduction. The extremes of abduction and internal rotation are best avoided in plaster due to the corresponding risk of avascular necrosis.

Following surgery computed tomography, magnetic resonance imaging or ultrasound should be used to confirm that the hip remains reduced. A hip spica cast should be maintained for three months. If during this time, it becomes evident that that the hip has dislocated in plaster then one should proceed to open reduction. Similarly, if one is unable to achieve a stable, congruent joint during closed reduction then one should proceed to open reduction.

Open reduction can be performed by either an anterolateral or medial approach. During open reduction, it is essential to identify and remove the thickened ligamentum teres as well as the fatty pulvinar. The hypertrophied transverse acetabular ligament and iliopsoas should be divided.

The advantage of an anterolateral approach is that most surgeons are familiar with it. It allows for good exposure and can be extended to allow for other procedures such as a pelvic osteotomy. However, as well as being associated with greater intra-operative bleeding than the alternative medial approaches it can damage the hip abductors.

The medial approaches to the hip carry the advantage of approaching the hip in line with the obstacles to reduction. However, it provides a comparatively poorer view of the hip joint and carries with it the possibility of injury to the medial circumflex femoral artery.

Similar to closed reduction, a hip spica cast is required for three months with reduction being confirmed intra operatively via radiographs and post operatively via computed tomography.

In the child older than two years, treatment is challenging and is very much based upon open reduction. Femoral shortening is also often required to lower the pressure upon the proximal femur and thus avoid proximal femoral growth disturbance.

For those between the ages of two and three years, there is only limited potential for acetabular remodelling and thus a pelvic procedure is often required in addition to an open reduction. The usual approach is to assess acetabular coverage during an open reduction. If it is insufficient, an osteotomy should be performed. If the hip appears stable, the acetabulum can simply be observed.

Should a pelvic osteotomy be required, it is usually a Salter or Pemberton osteotomy. A Salter osteotomy aims to improve coverage of the femoral head by moving acetabulum in an anterolateral direction. Pemberton's osteotomy improves anterolateral coverage of the femoral head.

## Complications

Avascular necrosis remains the most feared complication arising from the treatment of DDH. It arises due to too great a pressure being applied upon the femoral head. The position of immobilisation is of critical importance in preventing avascular necrosis. The extremes of abduction and internal rotation must be avoided. In the child, avascular necrosis can be diagnosed when the femoral head fails to grow after one year following reduction.

Degenerative joint disease also remains a feared complication. Those with untreated DH can develop arthritic changes in their hips by their thirties [24]. In adults, Crowe's classification is of use in describing DDH. It is divided into four groups with type 1 representing less than 50% subluxation, type 2 represents between 50 and 75% subluxation, type 3 represents between 75 and 100% subluxation while type 4 represents a dislocated hip. Type 2 and 3 hips are associated with premature arthritis whilst the dislocated hip's prognosis depends upon the presence or absence of a pseudoacetabulum. In those hips that are dislocated but without a pseudo-acetabulum, arthritis may not develop. Meanwhile, the dislocated hip that has a pseudo-acetabulum can have a range of presentations from minimal arthritis to significant degenerative changes. Ultimately, the degenerative hip may become symptomatic enough to require total hip arthroplasty or hip fusion surgery.

## Conclusion

DDH encompasses a spectrum of disease from minor dysplasia that resolves in the first few weeks of life to frank dislocation of hip. Well documented risk factors for DDH have been documented; neonates with a history of these risk factors should be carefully examined clinically for DDH. There may be a role for ultrasound screening in those with risk factors also. At any rate, all neonates should be screened for DDH via clinical examination. The case for universal screening has yet to be made principally due to the risks of overtreatment.

Ultrasound does, however, have a role in confirming a diagnosis of DDH as well as confirming reduction post treatment. Radiographs are not of use in the neonate but are helpful in the child over 6 months. An understanding of various reference lines is helpful in the interpretation of radiographs.

The ideal is for all cases to be identified at birth and for treatment to be instituted as is felt appropriate by the treating orthopaedic surgeon. In most cases, treatment will be delayed for 2 weeks in case the hip instability improves with age. If not, treatment with splintage is recommended in most cases. In the older child, closed or open reduction may well be required. In certain cases, open reduction may well need to be combined with pelvic procedures.

## References

[1] Taybi H, Lachman RS (1996). *Radiology of syndromes, metabolic disorders, and skeletal dysplasias* (4th edn). St. Louis: Mosby-Year Book.

[2] Soo B, Howard JJ, Boyd RN et al (2006) Hip displacement in cerebral palsy. *J. Bone. Joint. Surg. Am.,* 88A(1), 121–129.

[3] P. Klisic (1989). Congenital dislocation of the hip—a misleading term. *J. Bone. Joint. Surg. Br.,* 71, 136 – XXXX.

[4] Bjerkreim I, Arseth PH (1978). Congenital dislocation of the hip in Norway. Late diagnosis CDH in the years 1970 to 1974. *Acta. Paediatr. Scand.,* 67, 329–32.

[5] Haasbeek JF, Wright JG, Hedden DM (1995). Is there a difference between the epidemiologic characteristics of hip dislocation diagnosed early and late? *Can. J. Surg.,* 38, 437–8.

[6] Wilkinson JA (1972). A post-natal survey for congenital displacement of the hip. *J. Bone. Joint. Surg. Br.,* 54, 40–9.

[7] Salter RB (1968). Etiology, pathogenesis and possible prevention of congenital dislocation of the hip. *Can. Med. Assoc. J.,* 98, 933–45.

[8] Dormans JP (2005). *Pediatric orthopaedics: core knowledge in orthopaedics* (1st edn). Philadephia: Elsevier – Mosby.
[9] Leck I, Congenital dislocation of the hip (2000). In: Wald N, Leck I, (Eds). *Antenatal and neonatal screening* (2nd edn, 398–424), Oxford,Oxford University Press.
[10] Marks DS, Clegg J, Al-Chalabi AN (1994). Routine ultrasound screening for neonatal hip instability, *J. Bone. Joint. Surg. Br.* 76, 534–538.
[11] Ortolani M (1937). Un segno poco noto e sua importanza per la diagnosi precoce di prelussazione congenita dell'anca. *Pediatria* (Napoli), 45, 129–136.
[12] Barlow TG (1962). Early diagnosis and treatment of congenital dislocation of the hip. *J. Bone. Joint. Surg. Br.,* 44, 292–301.
[13] Bialik V, Fishman J, Katzir J, Zeltzer M (1986). Clinical assessment of hip instability in the newborn by an orthopedic surgeon and a paediatrician. *J. Pediatr. Orthop.,* 6, 703–705.
[14] El-Shazly M, Trainor B, Kernohan WG et al. (1994). Reliability of the Barlow and Ortolani tests for neonatal hip instability. *J. Med. Scr.* 1, 165–168.
[15] Jari S, Paton RW, Srinivasan MS (2002). Unilateral limitation of abduction of the hip. A valuable clinical sign for DDH? *J. Bone. Joint. Surg. Br.,* 84, 104–107.
[16] Graf R, Wilson B (1995). *Sonography of the infant hip and its therapeutic implications.* Weinheim: Chapman and Hall.
[17] Harcke HT, Clarke NM, Lee MS, Borns PF, MacEwen GD (1984). Examination of the infant hip with real-time ultrasonography. *J. Ultrasound Med.,* 3 ,131–137.
[18] Rosendahl K, Markestad T, Lie RT (1994). Ultrasound screening for developmental dysplasia of the hip in the neonate: the effect of treatment rate and prevalence of late cases. *Pediatrics;* 94, 47 – 52.
[19] Garn SM, Rohmann CG, Silverman FN (1967). Radiographic standards for postnatal ossification and tooth calcification. *Med. Radiogr. Photogr.,* 43(2), 45-66.
[20] Jones DA (1998). Neonatal detection of developmental dysplasia of the hip. *J. Bone. Joint. Surg. Br.,* 80, 943–945.
[21] Ganger R, Grill F, Leodolter S, Vitek M. Ultrasound screening of the neonatal hip: results and experiences. *Ultraschall Med.,* 12, 25–30.

[22] U. S. Preventive Services Task Force (2006). Screening for developmental dysplasia of the hip: recommendation statement. *Pediatrics,* 117, 898–902.

[23] Gardiner HM Dunn PM (1990). Controlled trial of immediate splinting versus ultrasonographic surveillance in congenitally dislocatable hips. *Lancet,* 336, 1553–1556.

[24] Hartofilakidis G, Karachalios T, Stamos KG (2000). Epidemiology, demographics, natural history of congenital hip disease in adults. *Orthopedics,* 23, 823–7.

In: Dysplasia
Editors: L. M. Sexton and H. J. Leach
ISBN 978-1-61942-600-9


*Chapter III*

# BONE DYSPLASIA: CAUSES, CLASSIFICATION AND TREATMENT OPTIONS

***Miguel Cantalejo Moreira*[*]*, Joaquín Casado Pardo and Patricia López Viejo***
Rheumatology Unit, Hospital Universitario de Fuenlabrada, Madrid, Spain

## ABSTRACT

Bone dysplasias are a large and heterogeneous group of entities with a monogenic origin, cause changes in growth and bone development. Can be monostotic or polyostotic, affecting different areas of the bone and causing complications in the short, medium and long term. Molecular biology techniques allow prenatal diagnosis can be supported by imaging techniques in utero. Currently there are two classifications are used: a radiological classification, developed in 2001, which includes 33 groups of dysplasia and 3 groups of dysostosis based on the commitment of bone segments. So that we can find metaphyseal, diaphyseal and epiphyseal bone dysplasia according to the affected bone segment in long bones. Spondylo bone dysplasia if there is commitment of the spine. O bone dysplasias affecting specific bones as the skull or clavicles. And another molecular classification, basis of genetic alteration, which consists of several groups depending on whether the defect causing the disease is

[*] E-mail: m.cantalejo@hotmail.com, m.cantalejo.hflr@salud.madrid.org, reumatologia.hflr@salud.madrid.org.

found in extracellular structural proteins, in metabolic pathways (ion channels, enzymes or transporters), in the folding and degradation of macromolecules or in the absence of proteoglycan degradation as in lysosomal diseases, in hormones or signal transduction mechanisms, in nuclear protein or transcription factors, in oncogenes and tumor suppressor genes or in metabolism and processing of DNA and RNA. Treatment options, as well as genetic counseling, are medical and surgical measures. They have no purpose but to support healing. In some types of bone dysplasia has recommended the use of bisphosphonates for prevention of vertebral fractures, remains controversial use of growth hormone.

Bone dysplasias are diseases of genetic origin, where a single gene is particularly impaired. Therefore, their origin is monogenic. The evolution of dysplasias is characterised by disorders in the development and growth of bone and cartilaginous tissue, eventually resulting in shape distortions and reduction in the size of the extremities, torso and/or skull. These entities can affect other organs, including: eye, congenital cataract or myopia; mouth, cleft palate; ear; central nervous system: hydrocephalus, agenesis of the corpus callosum and, in some cases, mental retardation; cardiovascular system: atrial septal defects, persistent ductus arteriosus, and large vessel transposition.

There are acquired forms of skeletal dysplasia, which occur more frequently than congenital forms. Neurological diseases associated with palsy may cause severe amyotrophy and secondary disorders in bone development and can eventually cause very fragile, dysplastic bones. Similarly, diseases involving prolonged bed confinement during growth can trigger the same disorders in the musculoskeletal system.

The main characteristic of bone dysplasias is low height, with three or more standard deviations below the mean height, for the age, sex and race of the patient. The incidence of these diseases is one per 3500/4000 newborns and is the cause of 2-3% of the complaints for low height in paediatrics.

The word dwarfing is a synonym of skeletal dysplasia, which means disproportionate short stature. It can affect the torso and the extremities. In the latter, they may be: rhizomelic, where the proximal part of the extremity is affected; mesomelic, involving the medial part of the extremity, and acromelic, where the distal part of the disease is involved. Other forms are to grow twisted dystrophy and camptomelic dystrophy, bent limbs.

Molecular biology techniques currently allow for prenatal diagnosis by cyto-genetic study of the amniotic fluid (amniocentesis) or chorionic villus (biopsy of chorionic villus), these techniques being supported by ultrasound evaluations.

In skeletal dysplasias, the most common type of inheritance is autosomal dominant. Autosomal recessive and sex-linked forms have been described, which are less common. Achondroplasia is the most common bone dysplasia. It occurs in 1 per 10000-15000 newborns. It originates in inborn errors in the growth cartilage. The gene affected is the fibroblastic growth factor receptor 3 (FGFR3), which is also the origin of thanatophoric dysplasia and hypochondroplasia. Other impaired genes are the origin of other dysplasias (Table 1). Therefore, in Schmid metaphyseal dysplasia, the gene COL10A1 is impaired, and in multiple epiphyseal dysplasia the gene COL9A2. Mutations of the COMP gene are the cause of 40% of the cases of pseudoachondroplasia. It must be stressed that a single gene can show several mutations and, therefore, can be the origin of several diseases. In this regard, the London Dismorphology Database (LDDB) describes that mutations in 40 genes are the origin of 104 different congenital diseases.

### Table I. Skeletal Dysplasias of Known Genetic Origin

1. Achondroplasia Group: Mutations in the fibroblast growth factor 3 gene FGFR3).
2. Diastrophic Dysplasia Group: Mutations in the diastrophic dysplasia sulfate transporter gene (DTDST).
3. Type II Collagenophaties: Mutations in the procollagen II gene (COL2A1).
4. Type XI Collagenophaties: Mutations in the procolagen XI gene (COL11A1 COL11A2).
5. Multiple Epiphyseal Dysplasia and Pseudoachondroplasia: Mutations in the cartilage oligomatrix protein gene (COMP).
6. Chondrodysplasia Punctata: Several Mutations:
   a) Arylsulfatase E gene (ARSE)
   b) X-lindked dominan chondrodysplasia Puntata Gene (CPXD)
   c) X-lindked recessive chondrodysplasia (CPDR)
   d) Genes responsible for production of the peroxisomal factors (PEX)
7. Metaphyseal Dysplasias: Three differents genetic mutations:
   a) Adenosine deaminase gene (ADA)
   b) The procollagen X gene (COL10A1)
   c) Gene responsible for parathyroid hormone- related polypeptide receptor (PTHR).
8. Acromelic and acromesomelicc Dysplasias: Genetic mutations in the genes responsible for encoding the cartilage-derived morphogenic protein-1-gene (CDMP1) and the guanine nucleotide-binding protein of the edenylate cyclase a-subunit. (GNAS-1).
9. Dysplasia with prominet membranous bone involvement: Mutation of the transcription core binding a 1-subunit gene. (CBFA1).
10. Bent-bone dysplasia group: Mutations in the SRY-box 9 protein (SOX-9).
11. Dysplasia whit defective mineralization: Several mutations:
    a) Liver alkaline phosphatase gene (ALPL)
    b) The parathyroid calcium-sensing receptor gene. (CASR)
    c) The X-Linked hypophosphatemia gene (PHEX)

There are forms of lethal skeletal dysplasias, that occur with a frequency of 1.5 per 10,000 births. The most common are osteogenesis imperfecta, thanatophoric dysplasia, achondrogenesis, and short rib polydactyly. In thanatophoric dysplasia, as in achondroplasia, disorders occur in the growth cartilage and they share the same gene in their origin: FGFR3. Osteogenesis imperfecta is caused by mutations in the type I collagen gene mutations: COL1A1 and COL1A2, yielding as a final result the disorganisation of the triple helix of type I collagen in the bone matrix. Achondrogenesis-hypochondrogenesis: Type I (Parenti-Fraccaro) and type II ( Langer-Saldino) are caused by changes in the type 2 collagen structure, by disorders in the secretion of bone matrix components, and by reduction in the production of decorin. All of this causes weakness and lack of integrity of the whole bone matrix.

## Classification of Bone Dysplasias

Skeletal dysplasias or osteochondrodysplasias are a clinically, phenotypically and genetically heterogeneous group of disorders involving the skeletal system and which arise through disturbances in the processes of skeletal development, growth and homeostasis. They have always been considered to be generalized disorders of endochondral and/or membranous ossification, their clinical and molecular heterogeneity is being elucidated.

Skeletal disorders have been divided into dysostoses, malformations of individual bones or groups of bones, which are caused by morphogenic embryonic defects. They arise from embryonic morphogenenic defects and are more closely related to multiple malformation syndromes. And osteochondrodysplasias, primary generalized developmental disorders and the growth of chondro-osseous tissue, which mainly occur in tubular bones and/or in the spine because of defects in structural proteins or metabolic procesess.

Individual skeletal dysplasias are quite rare but, as a group, they are more common and their clinical relevance, as one the main causes of a severe growth retardation, has a significant effect on morbidity and mortality at all ages.

Many attempts have been made to identify this diseases group in order to facilitate their diagnosis and to draw conclusions about possible underlying pathomechanisms. At present, there is no available a complete system of classification for genetic bone diseases. Due to the rarity of their individual qualities; their extensive heterogeneity, with more than 400 recognized forms of skeletal dysplasia currently; and their complex physiopathology; these entities pose a challenge in their study and their diagnosis.

At first, anathomic classifications were used, according to what was observed in the morphology. From this point of view and depending on the osseous part which is affected, these disorders can be classified as: rhizomelic, when the affected part is the proximal one: an arm or a thigh; mesomelic, which affects the medial osseous portions: a forearm or a leg; and acromelic, which affects the distal osseous portion: a hand or a foot. Combinations of the above mentioned types may also occur.

Later on, radiologic classifications started to be used. Nevertheless, molecular classification is more widely used on account of the developments on the field of genetics. Despite this fact, radiologic classification is still needed to differ among the various types of skeletal dysplasias.

The radiologic study is essential and allows to find out which is the role of certain bones and clarify which are the parts of the bones that are affected. Moreover, when the radiologic study is carried out, in addition to the alterations found predominant in epiphysis, diaphysis and metaphysis of tubular bones, not in combination with other bones, can also be found certain peculiar findings characteristic of osteochondrodysplasia, these findings are for instance:

- Bowing of long bones in the osteogenesis imperfecta and in the campomelic dysplasia.
- Epiphyseal calcifications in the congenital calcifying chondrodystrophy.
- Accentuated shortening of the ribs in the chondroectodermal dysplasia.
- Fractures of the tubular bones in the severe hypophosphatasia during the neonatal period.
- Lack of ossification of vertebral bodies in the achondrogenesis.
- Platyspondyly and/or segmentation of vertebral bodies in the thanatophoric dysplasia.

The degree of commitment of other bones in combination or not with the damage of long bones or with other bones, can be established through the radiologic study as is shown in the following cases:

- Spondylo dysplasia, which involves a commitment of the spine. Spondyloepiphyseal and spondylometaphyseal dysplasias when there is also commitment of the epiphysis and metaphysis, respectively.
- Craneometaphyseal or craneospondylometaphyseal dysplasia, which affect the skull and the metaphysis of long bones; or the skull, the metaphysis and the spine, respectively.
- Cleidocraneal dysplasia, when some particular bones are affected, such as the clavicle and the skull in this case.

Thus, radiologic classification is based on the commitment of different osseous segments, consequently we can find various types:

- Epiphyseal dysplasias, such as multiple epiphyseal dysplasia, dysplasia epiphysealis hemimelica and spondyloepiphseal dysplasia.
- Physeal dysplasias, as for example achondroplasia, hypochondroplasia and enchondromatosis or Ollier's disease.
- Metaphyseal dysplasias, which are subdivided into:

    - Hyperplasias, such as metaphyseal dysplasia or Pyles dysplasia, cranio-metaphyseal dysplasia and metaphyseal chondrodysplasia Jansen type, Schmid type, Spahr-Hartmann type and McKusick type.
    - Hypoplasias, such as the hypophosphatasia, osteopetrosis, hereditary exostosis, osteopathia striata, osteopoikilosis and melorrheostosis.

- Diaphyseal dysplasias, as osteogenesis imperfecta, from type I to type IV, progressive diaphyseal dysplasia or Engelmann's disease and craniodiaphyseal dysplasia.
- Other dysplasias or related conditions, such as diastrophic dwarfism, cleidocranial dysplasia, pyknodysostosis, fibrous dysplasias, fibrodysplasia or myositis ossificans progressive, nail patella syndrome, Marfan disease, homocystinuria, acrocephalosyndactyly or Aperts disease, Ehler's Danlos syndrome and the mucopolysaccharidosis, as type I or Hurlers disease, type II or Hunters syndrome, or type IV or Morquios disease.

The use of radiodiagnostics in the delineation of bone dysplasias is basically to distinguish between those lethal osteochondrodysplasias and the ones which are not so. Radiology meets its limits when different mutations lead to identical or overlapping phenotypes. Nowadays radiology keeps its prominent place in the diagnosis and nosology of inborn errors of skeletal development because of its ready availability, its speed, its non-invasiveness and its discriminating power. But where radiology is more important is in the evaluation of the prognosis of a particular entity.

Clinical manifestations and radiologic studies are fundamental for the differential diagnosis of skeletal dysplasias. Nevertheless, both prenatal and outright postpartum diagnoses are achieved by means of a genetic study. Clinical manifestations and radiological investigations are crucial for the differential diagnosis in skeletal dysplasias. However, prenatal diagnosis and postnatal definitive diagnosis are achieved by genetic study, which leads into a molecular-pathogenetic classification. Mutations responsible for these disorders may cause:

1) Qualitative or quantitative defects in the synthesis of structural extracellular proteins, as for example in the case of osteogenesis imperfecta, hypochondrogenesis, multiple epiphyseal dysplasia and pseudoachondroplasia.
2) Defects in the metabolic pathways, enzyme, ionic channels or transporters such as in the case of cranio-metaphyseal dysplasia, severe hypophosphatasia, and diastrophic dysplasia.
3) Defects in the folding, processing, transport and degradation of macromolecules such as in the case of mucopolysaccharidosis, piknodiostosis, types II and III of mucolipidosis and querubism.
4) Defects in hormones, factors of growth, mechanisms of transduction of signals and receivers, for instance craniosynostosis, thanatophoric dysplasia, achondroplasia and metaphyseal dysplasia.
5) Defects in nuclear proteins and factors of transcription, such as cleidocraneal dysplasia, camptomelic dysplasia and Turner's syndrome.
6) Defects in the processing and metabolism of RNA and DNA, such as in the case of cartilage-hair hypoplasia.
7) Defects in the proteins of the cytoskeleton, such as frontometaphyseal dysplasia.

8) Defects in identified responsible genes which have an unknown function, as in Smith McCort's syndrome; and defects in oncogenes and tumor supressor genes, as for example in multiple exotosis.

The number of recognized genetic disorders with a significant skeletal component is growing and the distinction between dysplasias, metabolic bone disorders, dysostoses, and malformation syndromes is blurring. That is why it is trying to create a classification where the molecular and pathogenic characteristics of the different entities are integrated with the clinic characteristics and their radiologic appearance. Molecular diagnosis does not only lead to the confirmation of single entities and the constititution of new groups of disorders, but it also allows the delimitation of entities that are related to each other, despite being different. This implies the heterogeneity of molecular mechanisms, as well as an incresase in the number of entities and their complexity. Therefore, this classification offers a view of recognized osseous disorders which are grouped according to their clinical, radiologic and molecular pathogenesis characteristics, whose goal would provide an updated vision of the medical-scientific community of those disorders with known bone component and their underlying genetic defects that can provide certain aid when diagnosing individual cases of genetic diseases of the skeleton, as well as helping with the recognition and delimitation of new entities which appear with the current development of the technology of sequences; and promote research in skeletal biology and related genetic disorders, looking for the clinical correlation between genes and proteins which are involved.

In the 60s, a Nosology and Classification of Genetic Disorders of the Skeleton was designed in order to cope with the huge amount of genetic disorders of bones which were clinically and genetically different, this Nosology has been revised and updated periodically by the members of the International Skeletal Dysplasia Society ( ISDS). The classification has evolved in the last 30 years, since it was publised for the first time in 1970. At first, it was based on the clinic and radiographic characteristics, later on biochemical and molecular characteristics were added, which are more appropriate to understand physiopathology and more useful in the recognition of metabolic pathways related to the development of the skeleton and those genes which are likely to be therapeutic target

That is the reason why the evaluation of these disorders requires a multidisciplinary approach involving many different specialists: clinical geneticists, molecular biologists, biochemists, radiologists, pediatricians, orthopedists and psychiatrists.

Especific genetic defects which underlay on many of these entities have been solved, this has allowed to establish links between the phenotype and the genotype and to be able to write an etiological classification of an increasing number of these osseous disorders. The previous versions of the classification of the genetic disorders of the skeleton have been based on the concept that similar phenotypically disorders would have coincidental molecular basis, due to the slight biochemical and molecular information which was available at that time. In fact, some groups of disorders are still defined taking into account their common radiographic characteristics or their anatomical location. This concept has been partly confirmed because of the identification of biochemically related groups and genetic families. However, more developments in the field of molecular genetics are proving that all this is not caused due to defects in genes or common physiological pathways. Important developments have been carried out on the identification of molecular changes which are resposible for the defined entities. Thus, new diseases are constantly being tracked down. The criteria used to include genetic disorders of bones in the classification are the ones which follow:

1) Significant skeletal involvement, corresponding to the definition of skeletal dysplasias, metabolic bone disorders, dysostoses, skeletal malformations and/or reduction syndromes.
2) Publication and /or listing in MIM.
3) Genetic basis proven or based on homogeneity of phenotype in unrelated families.
4) Nosologic autonomy confirmed by molecular or linkage analysis and/or by the presence of distinctive diagnostic features and of observation in multiple individuals or families.

Nosologic status of every disorder was classified as final, when there are mutations or identified locus; probable, when there are evidences; or bona fide, when there are multiple observations and clear diagnostic criteria, but there are still no evidences, nor identified locus.

Within a group, disorders with known molecular basis have been listed preceding those with lesser degree of evidence; however, variants of the same disorder have been kept together.

In the last revision in 2010, 456 different entities were included and placed in 40 groups defined by molecular, biochemical and/or radiographic criteria. Among these, 316 entities were associated with mutations in one or more of 226 different genes, going from common and recurrent mutations to specific mutations in concrete families or individuals.

Groups from 1 to 8 are based on a molecule, a gene or a common underlying pathway which is affected.

1) FGFR3 chondrodysplasia group
2) Type 2 collagen group and similar disorders
3) Type 11 collagen group
4) Sulfation disorders group
5) Perlecan group
6) Aggrecan group
7) Filamin group and related disorders
8) TRPV4 group

Groups from 9 to 17 are based on the locations of radiographic changes of specific osseous structures: epiphysis, metaphysis, diaphysis, vertebrae or a combination of them; or of the affected segment: rhizo, meso or acro.

9) Short-ribs dysplasias (with or without polydactyly) group
10) Multiple epiphyseal dysplasia and pseudoachondroplasia group.
11) Metaphyseal dysplasias
12) Spondylometphyseal dysplasias (SMD)
13) Spondylo-epi-(meta)-physeal dysplasias (SE(M)D)
14) Severe spondylodysplastic dysplasias)
15) Acromelic dysplasias
16) Acromesomelic dysplasias
17) Mesomelic and rhizo-mesomelic dysplasias

Groups from 18 to 20 are defined by macroscopic criteria which are combined with clinical characteristics: slender or bent bones, the presence of multiple disorders, etc.

18) Bent bones dysplasias
19) Slender bone dysplasia group
20) Dysplasias with multiple joint dislocations

Groups from 21 to 25 and group 28 are based on characteristics of mineralization: an increase or decrease of bone density, impaired mineralization, stippling or osteolysis. Moreover, the group of abnormal mineralization (group 26) involves different molecular mechanisms which lead to hypophosphatemic rickets. In the case of group 27 or multiple dysostosis, this is a wide group of lysosomal diseases which affect bones.

21) Chondrodysplasia punctata (CDP) group
22) Neonatal osteosclerotic displasias
23) Increased bone density group (without modification of bone shape)
24) Increased bone density group with metaphyseal and/or diaphyseal involvement
25) Osteogenesis imperfecta and decreased bone density group
26) Abnormal mineralization group
27) Lysosomal storage diseases with skeletal involvement (dysostosis multiplex group)
28) Osteolysis group

Group 29 is a very heterogeneous group, which includes those abnormal disorders produced by a disrupted development of the skeleton components. Group 30 involves disorders that show syndromes of overgrowth with significant bone involvement as part of the diagnostic criteria. Group 31 includes those disorders that show inflammatory characeristics or those which affect in a similar way to rheumatoid and genetically inflammatory osteoarthropathy.

29) Disorganized development of skeletal components group
30) Overgrowth lesyndromes with sketal involvement
31) Genetic inflammatory/rheumatoid-like osteoarthropathies

Groups from 32 to 40 involve dysostoses following anatomic criteria: skull, face, axial skeleton, extremities; and additional criteria which reflect the principles of embryonic development.

32) Cleidocranial dysplasia and isolated cranial ossification defects group
33) Craniosynostosis syndromes
34) Dysostoses with predominan craniofacial involvement

35) Dysostoses with predominant vertebral with and without costal involvement
36) Patellar dysostoses
37) Brachydactylies (with or without extraskeletal manifestations)
38) Limb hypoplasia—reduction defects group
39) Polydactyly–Syndactyly–Triphalangism group
40) Defects in joint formation and synostoses

The classification is a hybrid between a list of clinically defined disorders, with molecular clarifications that come up and a database which keeps record of the phenotypic spectrum in every entity, due to the mutations of a particular gene. Therefore, the first aim of the classification is to provide with a list of reference and the second objective is to help with the diagnosis, that is why it must coexist with some other classifications which are based on a clinical, radiologic or molecular approach.

## Treatment and Management of Skeletal Dysplasia

Treatment and management of children with skeletal dysplasia begins, in some cases, when child is born. Accurate diagnosis of skeletal dysplasia in children, particularly in newborn babies, while often challenging, is required to anticipate physical complications and provide appropriate genetic counselling. Diagnosis is based on clinical features, skeletal radiography and laboratory tests, specially genetic and metabolic studies. Many complications are common and require regular anticipatory assessment with implementation of appropriate intervention. Others are rarer but can cause significant morbidity; thus, specific surveillance is recommended for early detection. Although most individuals with skeletal dysplasia have a normal life expectancy, some bone dysplasia are lethal and sometimes neonatal resuscitation may be necessary for infants with more severe types of bone dysplasia, including thoracic cavity anomalies.

The medical management of children with bone dysplasia begins at birth and continues into adulthood. In children with achondroplasia excess weight gain is frequently a significant issue for many affected children. Maintaining an appropriate height and weight control from an early age will help avoiding long-term complications of this generalised skeletal disorder. Obesity is a risk for children with skeletal dysplasia. Excess weight can cause serious complications, including breathing difficulties such as sleep apnea, and may aggravate other, such as spinal cord compression and joint instability found in many types of bone dysplasia.

These patients often develop a thoracolumbar kyphosis that in the majority this will correct spontaneously. When the kyphosis not fully correct may be necessary referral to an orthopaedic surgeon.

Joint involvement as hypermobility is a very common feature of achondroplasia.

There are frecuently flexion contractures in elbows and hips. Physioterapy may improve hip flexion contractures and reduce the severity of symptoms related to spinal stenosis later in adulthood. The elbow contractures do not improve with physiotherapy.

Surgical treatment of skeletal dysplasia varies depending on the specific type present and the associated conditions. In some individuals with short-limbed types of skeletal dysplasia, lengthening of the limbs using surgical techniques based on distraction osteotomy has been successful. Extended limb lengthening is a multistage procedure, where long bones are fractured and then allowed to heal while external fixators apply traction as new bone forms, and has had a controversial history. The psychological assessment before surgery and the participation of the children in the decisions is very important.

Medical treatments include the administration of recombinant human growth hormone (hGH) has been shown variable results. This approach has been shown to be safe and effective for the treatment of short stature in various populations, including GH deficiency, small for gestacional age, Turner syndrome, Noonan syndrome, children receiving long-term glucocorticoid therapy, chronic renal insufficiency, and idiopathic short stature.

The growth of untreated children with achondroplasia is typical. Recombinant human growth hormone has been able to maintain growth in the 50 percentile using the hGH at a dose of 30-40 units/m$^2$/week. It should be administered early, and has been shown that the results are most effective when treatment is started before 2 years of age. Results from the ANSWER Program registry suggest that many patients start hGH treatment later than desirable; multiple studies suggest better growth outcomes with earlier intervention.

In summary, in the management of patients with bone dysplasia is very important that patients affected avoid excess weight gain and have joint hygienic measures, in order to prevent deformities and disabilities and improve quality of life in affected children and their families. Furthermore, some bone dysplasia are susceptible to specific treatments such as surgery or hormone growth that can improve the final prognosis.

## REFERENCES

[1] Goncalves L, Jeanty P. *Fetal biometry of skeletal dysplasia*. A multicentric study. J Ultrasoun Med 1994; 13: 977-85.

[2] International nomenclature and classification of the osteochondrodysplasias (1997). *International Working Group on Constitutional Diseases of Bone*. Am J Med Genet 1998; 79: 376-82.

[3] Maroteaux P. *International nomenclature of constitutional diseases of bones with bibliography*. Birth Defects Orig Artic Ser 1986; 22: 1-54.

[4] Sillence DO, Horton WA, Rimoin DL. *Morphologic studies in the skeletal dysplasias*. Am J Pathol 1979; 96: 813-70

[5] Francomano CA. *The genetic basis of dwarfism*. N Engl J Med 1995; 332: 58-9.

[6] Bonaventure J, Rousseau F, Legeai-Mallet L, Lr Merrer ML, Munnich A, Maroteaux P. *Common mutations in the fibroblast growth factor receptor 3 (FGFR3) gene account for achondroplasia, hypochondroplasia, and thanatophoric dwarfism*. Am J Med Genet 1996; 63: 148-54.

[7] Cole WG, Dalgleish R. *Perinatal lethal ostegenesis imperfecta*. J Med Genet 1995; 32: 284-9.

[8] Hortop J, Tsipouras P, Hanley JA, Maron BJ, Shapiro JR. *Cardiovascular involvement in osteogenesis imperfecta*. Circulation 1986; 73: 54-61.

[9] Hoefler S, Hoefler G, Moser A, Watkins P, Chen W, HW M. *Prenatal diagnosis of rhizomielic chondrodysplasia punctata*. Prenatal Diag 1988; 8: 571-6.

[10] Ascurra M, Herreros MB, Rodriguez S. *Displasias Óseas: a propósito de cuatro nosologías diferentes*. 2003; Available at: http://scielo.iics .una.py/pdf/iics/v1n1/v1n1a04.pdf. Accessed 8/10/2011, 2011.

[11] Azouz EM, Teebi AS, Eydoux P, Chen MF, Fassier F. *Bone dysplasias: an introduction*. Can Assoc Radiol J 1998 Apr;49(2):105-109.

[12] Chen H. *Skeletal Dysplasia Clinical Presentation*. 2009; Available at: http://emedicine.medscape.com/article/943343-clinical#a0218. Accessed 8/10/2011, 2011.

[13] Cortés F. *Displasias Esqueleticas.* 2006; Available at: http://www .acondroplasiauruguay.org/documentos/informacion%20medica/a/Displasias%20Esqueleticas%20Dra%20Fanny%20Cortes%20Chile.pdf. Accessed 8/10/2011, 2011.

[14] Despres S, Engel MW, Zabel B. *Skeletal dysplasias.* The network SKELNET. Bundesgesundheitsblatt Gesundheitsforschung Gesundheitsschutz 2007 Dec;50(12):1548-1555.

[15] Hall CM. *International nosology and classification of constitutional disorders of bone (2001).* Am J Med Genet 2002 Nov 15;113(1):65-77.

[16] Kornak U, Mundlos S. *Genetic disorders of the skeleton: a developmental approach.* Am J Hum Genet 2003 Sep;73(3):447-474.

[17] Lenz W. *Bone diseases: review and classification of congenital developmental disorders.* Monatsschr Kinderheilkd 1989 Aug;137 (8): 428-437.

[18] Namba N. *Genetic basis for skeletal disease. Nosology and molecular classification of skeletal dysplasias.* Clin Calcium 2010 Aug;20(8):1159-1165.

[19] Offiah AC, Hall CM. *Radiological diagnosis of the constitutional disorders of bone. As easy as A, B, C?* Pediatr Radiol 2003 Mar; 33 (3): 153-161.

[20] Orthopaedia Collaborative Orthopaedic Knowledgebase. *Bone Dysplasias.* 2010; Available at: http://www.orthopaedia.com /display /Review/Bone+Dysplasias. Accessed 8/10/2011, 2011.

[21] Rimoin DL, Cohn D, Krakow D, Wilcox W, Lachman RS, Alanay Y. *The skeletal dysplasias: clinical-molecular correlations.* Ann N Y Acad Sci 2007 Nov;1117:302-309.

[22] Sánchez Moreno EA. *Osteocondrodisplasia: una mirada a la acondroplasia.* 2010; Available at: http://www.acpp.com.co /web/index.php?option=com_content&view=article&id=17:osteocondrodisplasias&catid=31:ped-generales&Itemid=46. Accessed 8/10/2011, 2011.

[23] Savarirayan R, Rimoin DL. The skeletal dysplasias. Best Pract Res Clin Endocrinol Metab 2002 Sep;16(3):547-560.

[24] Spranger J. *Classification of skeletal dysplasias.* Acta Paediatr Scand Suppl 1991;377:138-142.

[25] Spranger J. *Radiologic nosology of bone dysplasias.* Am J Med Genet 1989 Sep;34(1):96-104.

[26] Superti-Furga A, Bonafe L, Rimoin DL. *Molecular-pathogenetic classification of genetic disorders of the skeleton.* Am J Med Genet 2001 Winter;106(4):282-293.

[27] Superti-Furga A, Unger S. *Nosology and classification of genetic skeletal disorders: 2006 revision.* Am J Med Genet A 2007 Jan 1;143(1):1-18.

[28] Tuysuz B. *A new concept of skeletal dysplasias*. Turk J Pediatr 2004 Jul-Sep;46(3):197-203.

[29] Warman ML, Cormier-Daire V, Hall C, Krakow D, Lachman R, LeMerrer M, et al. *Nosology and classification of genetic skeletal disorders: 2010 revision.* Am J Med Genet A 2011 May;155A(5):943-968.

[30] Rimoin David, Ralph Lachman, and Sheila Unger, *"Chrondfrodysplasia".* In Emery and Rimion´s Principles and Practice of Medical Genetics, 4th edition, edited by David L. Rimoin, J.Michael Connor, Reed Pyeritz, and Bruce R. Korf.London: Churchill Livingstone, 2002.

[31] Wright MJ, Irving MD.*Clinical management of achondroplasia*. Arch Dis Child (2011) Apr 3.

[32] González -Meneses López A. *Diagnostic orientation when bone dysplasia is suspected.* Pediatr Integral 2010; XIV (8):627-635.

[33] Ross J, Lee P.A, Gut R, Germak J. *Factors influencing the one-and two-year growth response in children treated with growth hormone: Analysis from an observational study.* International Journal of Pediatric Endocrynology 2010, Article ID 494656, 7 pages.

[34] Polgren L.E, Miller B.S. *Growth patterns and the use of growth hormone in the mucoplysaccharidoses*. J Pediatr Rehabil Med 2010 April 19;3(1): 25-38.

[35] Piana Román.A. *Displasias óseas*. Vol. 4 Número 1. Enero-Abril 2009 pp 5-9.

In: Dysplasia
Editors: L. M. Sexton and H. J. Leach
ISBN 978-1-61942-600-9


*Chapter IV*

# DOES ELEVATED INTRACELLULAR CHLORIDE CAUSE EPILEPSY IN FOCAL CORTICAL DYSPLASIA?

***Chigusa Shimizu-Okabe*[1]*, Akihito Okabe*[2] *and Atsuo Fukuda*[3]**

[1]Laboratory of Pharmacology,
Faculty of Pharmaceutical Sciences at Kagawa Campus,
Tokushima Bunri University, Sanuki, Kagawa, Japan
[2]Division of Physiome, Department of Physiology,
Hyogo College of Medicine, Nishinomiya, Hyogo, Japan
[3]Department of Physiology, Hamamatsu University School of Medicine,
Hamamatsu, Shizuoka, Japan

## ABSTRACT

γ-Aminobutyric acid (GABA) is the principal inhibitory neurotransmitter in the brain, and conventional anticonvulsant drugs often target the $GABA_A$ receptor chloride channel. However, GABA can become excitatory when intracellular chloride concentrations ($[Cl^-]_i$) are high. Depolarizing actions of GABA are seen not only in early development, but also in various pathological conditions. Cation-$Cl^-$ cotransporters play critical roles in the regulation of $[Cl^-]_i$. Extrusion of $Cl^-$ from cells is achieved by $K^+$-$Cl^-$cotransporters (KCCs), whereas $Na^+$-$K^+$-$2Cl^-$cotransporters (NKCCs) promote intracellular accumulation of $Cl^-$

. So far, at least four different mammalian subtypes of KCCs (KCC1-4) and two different subtypes of NKCCs (NKCC1-2) have been sequenced. Of these, KCC2 is present only in neurons while NKCC1 is expressed at moderate levels in both neurons and glial cells in the normal adult brain (Kanaka et al. 2001). In an animal model of epilepsy, NKCC1 expression has been found to be increased, while KCC2 mRNA was decreased in the hippocampus. Such changes in NKCC1 and/or KCC2 could lead to elevated $[Cl^-]_i$, and thereby cause an impairment in GABA-mediated inhibition. We have recently reported that KCC2 mRNA and protein levels were reduced in small neurons located around large abnormal neurons (giant cells) in human focal cortical dysplasia (FCD). However, NKCC1 expression did not differ among these cell types. These results indicate that downregulation of KCC2 may play a key role in the onset of seizures in FCD. Thus, high $[Cl^-]_i$ may play a role in inducing epilepsy in the human brain, through changes in $Cl^-$ regulation by KCC2 and NKCC1.

## INTRODUCTION

It has been proposed that an imbalance between excitatory and inhibitory synaptic transmission, in favor of excitation, leads to the initiation of epileptic discharges.GABA is the principal inhibitory neurotransmitter in the adult brain. GABA elicits hyperpolarizing responses via activation of the $GABA_A$ receptor chloride channel complex. Therefore, conventional anticonvulsant drugs, for example phenobarbital, often target the $GABA_A$ receptor.

Focal cortical dysplasia (FCD) is a well-recognized cause of pharmacoresistant epilepsy (Palmini et al. 1991, Raymond et al. 1995, Guerrini et al. 1999), and is characterized by a spectrum of histological features, including disorganization of cortical architecture with cells of abnormal size and polarity.The development of MRI techniques has facilitated the identification of FCD in patients with epilepsy. The epileptic focus can be removed by surgery (Sisodiya 2004, Kuzniecky and Barkovich 2001). The use of brain tissue taken from patients with FCD and animal models of epilepsy has contributed to an increasing understanding of epileptiform changes in GABAergic action, from hyperpolarizing to depolarizing. Because high $[Cl^-]_i$ causes depolarizing actions of GABA (Payne et al. 2003), $Cl^-$ homeostasis could be a very important factor in determining GABA function. This chapter will focus on the relationship between $Cl^-$ homeostatic changes in FCD and GABAergic depolarization, and the implications for anticonvulsant treatment will be discussed.

## GABA CAN BE BOTHINHIBITORY ANDEXCITATORY

The $[Cl^-]_i$ determines whether $GABA_A$ receptor activation causes hyperpolarization or depolarization.Cation-$Cl^-$cotransporters (CCCs) are well known to be critical for the normal regulation of $[Cl^-]_i$(Payne et al. 2003). The members of the CCC family show different patterns of tissue expression and perform a wide variety of physiological roles. The CCC family has large N- and C- terminal tails and 12 transmembrane domains. $K^+$-$Cl^-$cotransporters (KCCs) appear to mainly extrude $Cl^-$ from cells, whereas $Na^+$-$K^+$-$2Cl^-$ cotransporters (NKCCs) promote accumulation of intracellular $Cl^-$. So far, at least four different subtypes of KCCs (KCC1-4)and two NKCC subtypes (NKCC1-2)have been sequenced from mammals(Payne et al. 2003). KCC1-4 and NKCC1 are expressed in the brain, while the NKCC2 is predominantly expressed in the kidney. Of these, two cation-chloride cotransporters, KCC2 and NKCC1, may be of particular importance in controlling neural $Cl^-$ homeostasis(Payne et al. 1996, Rivera et al. 1999, Yamada et al. 2004). KCC2 is expressed only in neurons, and has two isoforms with different N termini, KCC2a and b (Uvarov et al. 2007). The NKCC1 can be found both in neurons and astrocytes (Kanaka et al. 2001, Hubner et al. 2001, Yan et al. 2001), and has two isoforms, NKCC1a and b. NKCC1a has a specific 16-amino acid domain encoded by exon 21 that contains a protein kinase A(PKA) phosphorylation site (Vibat et al. 2001).

GABAergic transmission is depolarizing during early development due to differential regulation of $Cl^-$ homeostasis (Ben-Ari et al.1989, Luhmann and Prince 1991, van den Pol 1996). The ontogeny of $Cl^-$ homeostasis is regulated by the differential expression of NKCC1 and KCC2 (Clayton et al. 1998, Shimizu-Okabe et al., 2002; Ikeda et al., 2003, Wang et al. 2002, Yamada et al. 2004). KCC2 shows a developmental increase whereas NKCC1 expression levels decrease after birth. Similarly, high NKCC1 levels and low KCC2 neuronal expression occurs in the immature human cortex (Dzhala et al. 2005, Aronica et al. 2007). The $[Cl^-]_i$of immature neurons is typically in the range of 25-40 mM in the rat brain (Achilles et al. 2007, Kakazu et al. 1999, Kilb et al. 2002, Yamada et al. 2004, Balakrishnan et al. 2003), whereas in mature neurons, the $[Cl^-]_i$ is typically ~5 mM (Yamada et al. 2004, Tyzio et al. 2008, Khirug et al. 2008). These developmental changes in $[Cl^-]_i$may be important in neocortical development, by modulating processes such as laminar organization and synaptogenesis (Ben-Ari, 2002).

Neuronal insults such as trauma or nerve axotomy are known to inducefunctional alterations in $Cl^-$ homeostasis (Nabekuraet al. 2002, Ueno et al. 2002, Toyoda et al.2003, Yan et al. 2001).For instance, NKCC1 protein expression increased in the cortex in response to ischemia (Yan et al. 2001), and treatment with the NKCC1 inhibitor bumetanide decreased the volume of a cortical infarct (Yan et al. 2001). On the other hand, peripheral nerve injury induced a downregulation of KCC2 expression and an increase in $[Cl^-]_i$ in lamina I neurons of the spinal cord (Coull et al. 2003). In addition, the expression of KCC2 mRNA was also downregulated by axotomy of the facial nerve. In this study, the resting $[Cl^-]_i$ of axotomized neurons wasaround 24 mM, which was significantly higher than that of intact neurons (11 mM)(Toyoda et al. 2003). Such dynamic changes of $Cl^-$ homeostasis by alterations in$Cl^-$cotransporter expression can reverse the action of GABA from hyperpolarizing to depolarizing.

## GABAergic Action Is Depolarizing in FCD

What about GABAergic function in FCD? Neurotransmission mediated by $GABA_A$ receptors did not seem to suppress epileptic discharges in pathological tissue (Avoli et al. 2005, Kohling et al. 1998). While a decreased immunoreactivity for $GABA_A$ receptor subunits has been reported in FCD tissue (Crino et al. 2001), changes in $GABA_A$ receptor expression alonecannot explain the mechanism of epileptogenesis in FCD.

In human FCD tissue, dysplastic neurons exhibited enhanced excitability and spontaneous seizure-like discharges (Avoli et al. 1999). Moreover, epileptic discharges in the human cortex with focal malformation were shown to be initiated by a synchronizing mechanism that relied on depolarizing GABA actions (D'Antuono et al. 2004). Neurons from individuals with adult FCD who have intractable seizures accumulate $Cl^-$ such that $GABA_A$ receptor activation is excitatory (Cohen et al. 2002, Huberfeld et al. 2007). Thus, $GABA_A$ receptor-mediated responses may change from hyperpolarizing to depolarizing in FCD tissue.

## CHLORIDE COTRANSPORTERS IN HUMAN FOCAL CORTICAL DYSPLASIA

Recent studies have investigated $Cl^-$ transporter levels in human epileptic tissue (Shimizu-Okabe et al. 2011, Aronicaet al.2007, Munakata et al. 2007, Muñoz et al.2007, Sen et al. 2007). Sen et al. (2007) showed that NKCC1 protein expression levels were increased in FCD, and Muñoz et al. (2007) reported a decrease in KCC2-immunoreactive neurons in hippocampal sclerosis. Some types of FCD are accompanied by disorganization of cortical architecture with cells of abnormal size and polarity (Palmini et al. 2004).Dysmorphic neurons are misshapen cells with abnormal orientation, size, structure and dendritic processes (Palmini et al. 2004). Balloon cells are abnormal cellular elements with thin membranes (Palmini et al. 2004). Immunoreactivity for KCC2 has been observed in neurons of different sizes, including large dysplastic neurons; however, KCC2 expression was not detected in balloon cells (Aronica et al. 2007, Munakata et al. 2007). Moreover, we recently reported that KCC2 mRNA and protein were expressed not only in non-dysplastic neurons in histologically normal portions located in the periphery of the excised cortex, but also in dysplastic cells in FCD tissue (Shimizu-Okabe et al. 2011). Compared with non-dysplastic neurons,KCC2 expression was significantly reduced in neurons located around large abnormal neurons, but not in the abnormal neurons themselves. The neurons located around large abnormal neurons were significantly smaller than non-dysplastic neurons.Downregulation of KCC2 and/or upregulation of NKCC1 could thus cause epileptogenesis.These findings indicate that human dysplastic tissue may retain immature properties, displaying mechanisms of seizure generation similar to those observed during development (Dzhala et al. 2005, Avoli et al. 2005).

In addition, Munakata et al. (2007) and Aronica et al. (2007) demonstrated a decrease in KCC2 protein expression and aberrant subcellular KCC2 localization in human cortical dysplasia. Taken together, these reports indicate that FCD may be accompanied by abnormalities in posttranslational modification of the KCC2 protein, leading to dysfunction of Cl- homeostasis. Posttranslational modification of the KCC2 protein is necessary for its membrane translocation and proper function (Wake et al. 2007, Lee et al. 2007). Lee et al. (2007) identified the protein residues involved in tyrosine phosphorylation of the KCC2 protein. KCC2 phosphorylation decreased the cell surface stability of the protein by enhancing lysosomal degradation (Wake et al. 2007, Lee et al. 2007).

## CHLORIDE HOMEOSTASIS IN ANIMAL MODELS OF EPILEPSY AND CHLORIDE COTRANSPORTER KNOCK-OUT MICE

Downregulation of KCC2 and/or upregulation of NKCC1 have been reported in animal models of epilepsy, and the results are similar to human cortical dysplasia. The expression levels of NKCC1 mRNA were increased in the piriform cortex and dentate gyrus following amygdala kindling (Okabe et al. 2002, 2003). KCC2 mRNA was downregulated in the mouse hippocampus after kindling-induced seizures (Rivera et al. 2002). Rivera et al. (2002) reported that KCC2 downregulation was mediated by molecular cascades involving brain-derived neurotrophic factor (BDNF)-TrkBsignaling.In the pilocarpine model of temporal lobe epilepsy, a shift in GABA equilibrium potential ($E_{GABA}$) is temporally restricted to the period of epileptogenesis, and has been suggested as a mechanism linking injury to the subsequent development of epilepsy (Pathak et al. 2007).

A pathological replay of a developmental process may thus be responsible for epileptogenesis in some cases (Cohen et al. 2003). Indeed, in an animal model of cortical malformation showing hyperexcitability (Jacobs et al. 1999), KCC2 downregulationand NKCC1 upregulationassociated with $[Cl^-]_i$ increases was found during formation of microgyri (Shimizu-Okabe et al. 2007, Sugimoto et al. 2003).

A genetic lack of KCC2 increases the susceptibilityto seizures. Double-deficient mice of KCC2a/b die within 24 hours after birth due to respiratory failure (Hübner et al. 2001). KCC2b-deficient mice exhibit frequent generalized seizures (Woo et al. 2002), andhypomorphic mice ($KCC2^{hy/null}$)which express ~17% of normal KCC2 (KCC2a and b) show increased seizure susceptibility (Tornberg et al. 2005). $E_{GABA}$ is about 20 mV more positive in $KCC2^{hy/null}$ mice than in wild-type animals (Riekki et al. 2008). These results suggest that the downregulation of KCC2 and/or upregulation of NKCC1 are associated with epileptogenesis.

## POSSIBLE THERAPIES FOR EPILEPSIES INDUCED BY ELEVATED INTRACELLULAR CHLORIDE

Barbiturates and benzodiazepines are used as anticonvulsant drugs to increase the effects of GABA. Phenobarbital is the drug of the first choice for

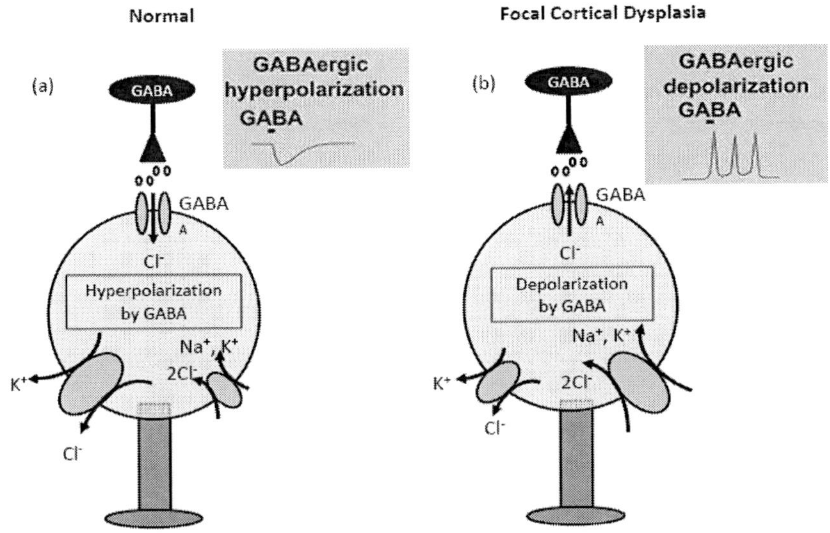


Figure. Schematic illustration of the proposed mechanisms of GABA action on seizures.

(a) GABA release from interneurons activates postsynaptic $GABA_A$ receptor chloride channels on cortical output neurons. This GABAergic action is hyperpolarizing in the normal adult brain because cortical neurons have low concentrations of intracellular $Cl^-$. The $Na^+$-$K^+$-$2Cl^-$cotransporter (NKCC1) mediates $Cl^-$ uptake, whereas the $K^+$-$Cl^-$ cotransporter (KCC2) extrudes $Cl^-$.NKCC1 expression is low, whereas the level of KCC2 expression is high.

(b) In focal cortical dysplasia, NKCC1 expression is increased and/or the level of KCC2 expression is decreased. The cortical neurons have a high concentration of $Cl^-$, rendering the $Cl^-$ equilibrium potential positive to the resting membrane potential. $GABA_A$ receptor chloride channel activation therefore results in $Cl^-$ efflux and a depolarizing action of GABA.

the therapy of neonatal seizures (Wheless et al. 2007, Bassan et al. 2008). These drugs only suppress the motor components of neonatal seizures, but have no effect on EEG seizures.

Neonatal seizures are difficult to treat. During early development, GABA produces excitatory responses in cortical neurons due to high $[Cl^-]_i$ (Luhmann and Prince 1991, Ben-Ari et al. 1989). NKCC1 is highly expressed in the rat and human cortex in the first two weeks after birth and then begins to decrease (Wang et al. 2003, Shimizu-Okabe et al.2003, Yamada et al. 2004, Dzhala et al. 2005). The expression of KCC2, on the other hand, increases one week after birth in rat and human cortex (Shimizu-Okabe et al. 2002, Dzhala et al. 2005). Consistent with this, Dzhala et al. (2005) showed that inhibition of

NKCC1 by bumetanide, which is used widely as a diuretic drug, suppressed kainate-induced seizures *in vivo*. Bumetanide also inhibited seizure-induced neonatal $Cl^-$ accumulation (Dzhala et al. 2005), and blocked spontaneous epileptiform bursts in the human adult epileptic subiculum (Huberfeld et al. 2007). Dzhala etal. (2010) recently reported efficacy of bumetanide in human neonatal seizure.

These reports provide evidence that inhibitors of CCCs may be useful for the treatment of seizures. However, because the diuretic drugs also affect transporters in thekidney, it may be necessary to develop the specific drugs for brain $Cl^-$cotransporters in the near future.

## REFERENCES

Achilles K, Okabe A, Ikeda M, Shimizu-Okabe C, Yamada J, Fukuda A, Luhmann HJ, Kilb W. Kinetic properties of Cl uptake mediated by Na+-dependent K+-2Cl cotransport in immature rat neocortical neurons. *J. Neurosci.* 2007, 27, 8616-27.

Aronica E, Boer K, Redeker S, Spliet WG, van Rijen PC, Troost D, Gorter JA. Differential expression patterns of chloride transporters, $Na^+$-$K^+$-$2Cl^-$ -cotransporter and $K^+$-$Cl^-$-cotransporter, in epilepsy-associated malformations of cortical development. *Neuroscience,* 2007, 145, 185-196.

Avoli M, Bernasconi A, Mattia D, Olivier A, Hwa GG. Epileptiform discharges in the human dysplastic neocortex: in vitro physiology and pharmacology. *Ann. Neurol.,* 1999, 46, 816-26.

Avoli M, Louvel J, Pumain R, Köhling R. Cellular and molecular mechanisms of epilepsy in the human brain. *Prog. Neurobiol.,* 2005, 77, 166-200

Balakrishnan V, Becker M, Löhrke S, Nothwang HG, Güresir E, Friauf E. Expression and function of chloride transporters during development of inhibitory neurotransmission in the auditory brainstem. *J. Neurosci.,* 2003, 23, 4134-45.

Ben-Ari, Y., Excitatory actions of GABA during development: the nature of the nurture. *Nat. Rev. Neurosci.*, 2002, 3, 728-739

Ben-Ari Y, Cherubini E, Corradetti R, Gaiarsa JL.,Giant synaptic potentials in immature rat CA3 hippocampal neurons. *J. Physiol.,* 1989,416, 303-325

Ben-Ari Y, Cherubini E, Corradetti R, Gaiarsa JL.Giant synaptic potentials in immature rat CA3 hippocampal neurons. *J. Physiol.* 1989, 416, 303-25

Clayton GH, Owens GC, Wolff JS, Smith RL.Ontogeny of cation-Cl- cotransporter expression in rat neocortex. *Brain Res. Dev. Brain Res.,* 1998, 109, 281-92.

Cohen I, Navarro V, Clemenceau S, Baulac M, Miles R. On the origin of interictal activity in human temporal lobe epilepsy in vitro. *Science,* 2002, 298, 1418-21.

Cohen I, Navarro V, Le Duigou C, Miles R. Mesial temporal lobe epilepsy: a pathological replay of developmental mechanisms? *Biol. Cell,* 2003, 95, 329-33.

Coull JA, Boudreau D, Bachand K, Prescott SA, Nault F, Sík A, De Koninck P, De Koninck Y.Trans-synaptic shift in anion gradient in spinal lamina I neurons as a mechanism of neuropathic pain. *Nature*, 2003, 424, 938-42.

Crino PB, Duhaime AC, Baltuch G, White R. Differential expression of glutamate and GABA-A receptor subunit mRNA in cortical dysplasia. *Neurology,* 2001, 56, 906-13.

D'Antuono M, Louvel J, Köhling R, Mattia D, Bernasconi A, Olivier A, Turak B, Devaux A, Pumain R, Avoli M. $GABA_A$ receptor-dependent synchronization leads to ictogenesis in the human dysplastic cortex. *Brain,* 2004, 127, 1626-40.

Dzhala VI, Talos DM, Sdrulla DA, Brumback AC, Mathews GC, Benke TA, Delpire E, Jensen FE, Staley KJ. NKCC1 transporter facilitates seizures in the developing brain. *Nat. Med.,* 2005, 11, 1205-13.

Dzhala VI, Kuchibhotla KV, Glykys JC, Kahle KT, Swiercz WB, Feng G, Kuner T, Augustine GJ, Bacskai BJ, Staley KJ. Progressive NKCC1-dependent neuronal chloride accumulation during neonatal seizures. *J. Neurosci.*, 2010, 30, 11745-61.

Fukuda A. Diuretic soothes seizures in newborns. *Nat. Med.* 2005, 11, 1153-54.

Guerrini R, Andermann E, Avoli M, Dobyns WB. Cortical dysplasias, genetics, and epileptogenesis. *Adv. Neurol.,* 1999, 79, 95-121.

Huberfeld G, Wittner L, Clemenceau S, Baulac M, Kaila K, Miles R, Rivera C. Perturbed chloride homeostasis and GABAergic signaling in human temporal lobe epilepsy. *J. Neurosci.* 2007, 27, 9866-73

Hübner CA, Stein V, Hermans-Borgmeyer I, Meyer T, Ballanyi K, Jentsch TJ.

Disruption of KCC2 reveals an essential role of K-Cl cotransport already in early synaptic inhibition. *Neuron,* 2001, 30, 515-24.

Ikeda M, Toyoda H, Yamada J, Okabe A, Sato K, Hotta Y, Fukuda A. Differential development of cation-chloride cotransporters and Cl- homeostasis contributes to differential GABAergic actions between developing rat visual cortex and dorsal lateral geniculate nucleus. *Brain Res.,* 2003, 984,149-59.

Jacobs KM, Hwang BJ, Prince DA. Focal epileptogenesis in a rat model of polymicrogyria. *J. Neurophysiol.,* 1999, 81, 159-73.

Kakazu Y, Akaike N, Komiyama S, Nabekura J.Regulation of intracellular chloride by cotransporters in developing lateral superior olive neurons. *J. Neurosci.,* 1999,19, 2843-51.

Kanaka C, Ohno K, Okabe A, Kuriyama K, Itoh T, Fukuda A, Sato K, The differential expression patterns of messenger RNAs encoding K-Clcotransporters (KCC1,2) and Na-K-2Cl cotransporter (NKCC1) in the rat nervous system. *Neuroscience,* 2001, 104, 933-46

Khirug S, Yamada J, Afzalov R, Voipio J, Khiroug L, Kaila K. GABAergic depolarization of the axon initial segment in cortical principal neurons is caused by the Na-K-2Cl cotransporter NKCC1. *J. Neurosci.* 2008 , 28, 4635-9.

Kilb W, Ikeda M, Uchida K, Okabe A, Fukuda A, Luhmann HJ. Depolarizing glycine responses in Cajal-Retzius cells of neonatal rat cerebral cortex. *Neuroscience,* 2002, 112, 299-307.

Köhling R, Lücke A, Straub H, Speckmann EJ, Tuxhorn I, Wolf P, Pannek H, Oppel F.Spontaneous sharp waves in human neocortical slices excised from epileptic patients. *Brain,* 1998, 121, 1073-87.

Kuzniecky RI, Barkovich AJ.Malformation of cortical development and epilepsy. *Brain Development,* 2001, 23, 2-11.

Lee HH, Walker JA, Williams JR, Goodier RJ, Payne JA, Moss SJ. Direct protein kinase C-dependent phosphorylation regulates the cell surface stability and activity of the potassium chloride cotransporter KCC2. *J. Biol. Chem.* 2007, 282, 29777- 29784.

Luhmann HJ, Prince DA. Postnatal maturation of the GABAergic system in rat neocortex. *J. Neurophysiol.,* 1991, 65 ,247-63.

Munakata M, Watanabe M, Otsuki T, Nakama H, Arima K, Itoh M, Nabekura J, Iinuma K, Tsuchiya S. Altered distribution of KCC2 in cortical dysplasia in patients with intractable epilepsy. *Epilepsia,* 2007, 48, 837-44.

Muñoz A, Méndez P, DeFelipe J, Alvarez-Leefmans FJ.Cation-chloride cotransporters and GABA-ergic innervation in the human epileptic hippocampus. *Epilepsia,* 2007, 48, 663-73.

Nabekura J, Ueno T, Okabe A, Furuta A, Iwaki T, Shimizu-Okabe C, Fukuda A, Akaike N. Reduction of KCC2 expression and GABAA receptor-mediated excitation after in vivo axonal injury. *J. Neurosci.,* 2002, 22, 4412-17.

Okabe A, Ohno K, Toyoda H, Yokokura M, Sato K, Fukuda A. Amygdala kindling induces upregulation of mRNA for NKCC1, a Na(+), K(+)-2Cl(-) cotransporter, in the rat piriform cortex. *Neurosci. Res.,* 2002, 44, 225-29.

Okabe A, Yokokura M, Toyoda H, Shimizu-Okabe C, Ohno K, Sato K, Fukuda A. Changes in chloride homeostasis-regulating gene expressions in the rat hippocampus following amygdala kindling. *Brain Res.,* 2003, 990, 221-26.

Palmini A, Andermann F, Olivier A, Tampieri D, Robitaille Y. Focal neuronal migration disorders and intractable partial epilepsy: results of surgical treatment. *Ann. Neurol.,* 1991, 30, 750-7.

Palmini A, Najm I, Avanzini G, Babb T, Guerrini R, Foldvary-Schaefer N, Jackson G, Lüders HO, Prayson R, Spreafico R, Vinters HV.Terminology and classification of the cortical dysplasias. *Neurology,* 2004, 62, S2-8.Review.

Pathak HR, Weissinger F, Terunuma M, Carlson GC, Hsu FC, Moss SJ, Coulter DA. Disrupted dentate granule cell chloride regulation enhances synaptic excitability during development of temporal lobe epilepsy. *J. Neurosci.,* 2007, 27, 14012-22.

Payne JA, Rivera C, Voipio J, Kaila K. Cation-chloride co-transporters in neuronal communication, development and trauma. *Trends in Neurosci.,* 2003, 26, 199-206.

Payne JA, Stevenson TJ, Donaldson LF. Molecular characterization of a putative K-Clcotransporter in rat brain.A neuronal-specific isoform. *J. Biol. Chem.,* 1996, 271, 16245-452.

Raymond AA, Fish DR, Sisodiya SM, Alsanjari N, Stevens JM, Shorvon SD. Abnormalities of gyration, heterotopias, tuberous sclerosis, focal cortical dysplasia, microdysgenesis, dysembryoplastic neuroepithelial tumour and dysgenesis of the archicortex in epilepsy. Clinical, EEG and neuroimaging features in 100 adult patients. *Brain,* 1995, 118, 629-60.

Riekki R, Pavlov I, Tornberg J, Lauri SE, Airaksinen MS, Taira T. Altered synaptic dynamics and hippocampal excitability but normal long-term plasticity in mice lacking hyperpolarizing GABA A receptor-mediated inhibition in CA1 pyramidal neurons. *J. Neurophysiol.,* 2008, 99,3075-89.

Rivera C, Li H, Thomas-Crusells J, Lahtinen H, Viitanen T, Nanobashvili A, Kokaia Z, Airaksinen MS, Voipio J, Kaila K, Saarma M.BDNF-induced TrkB activation down-regulates the K+-Cl- cotransporter KCC2 and impairs neuronal Cl- extrusion. *J. Cell Biol.,* 2002, 159, 747-752.

Rivera C, Voipio J, Payne JA, Ruusuvuori E, Lahtinen H, Lamsa K, Pirvola U, Saarma M, Kaila K. The $K^+/Cl^-$ co-transporter KCC2 renders GABA hyperpolarizing during neuronal maturation. *Nature,* 1999, 397, 251-55.

Sen A, Martinian L, Nikolic M, Walker MC, Thom M, Sisodiya SM. Increased NKCC1 expression in refractory human epilepsy. *Epilepsy Res.* 2007, 74, 220-27.

Shimizu-Okabe C, Okabe A, Kilb W, Sato K, Luhmann HJ, Fukuda A. Changes in the expression of cation-$Cl^-$ cotransporters, NKCC1 and KCC2, during cortical malformation induced by neonatal freeze-lesion. *Neurosci. Res.,* 2007, 59, 288-95.

Shimizu-Okabe C, Yokokura M, Okabe A, Ikeda M, Sato K, Kilb W, Luhmann HJ, Fukuda A. Layer-specific expression of Cl- transporters and differential [Cl-]i in newborn rat cortex. *Neuroreport,* 2002, 13, 2433-7.

Shimizu-Okabe C, Tanaka M, Matsuda K, Mihara T, Okabe A, Sato K, Inoue Y, Fujiwara T, Yagi K, Fukuda A. KCC2 was downregulated in small neurons localized in epileptogenic human focal cortical dysplasia. *Epilepsy Res.,* 2011, 93, 177-84.

Sisodiya SM. Surgery for focal cortical dysplasia. *Brain,* 2004, 127, 2383-2384.

Sugimoto M, Yamada J, Kilb W, Ueno S, Luhmann HJ, Fukuda, A.Regaining of GABA- and glycine-induced calcium influxes during formation of the microgyrus in an experimental model of cortical malformations. *Soc. Neurosci. Abstr.* 2003, 29, 888.9.

Tornberg J, Voikar V, Savilahti H, Rauvala H, Airaksinen MS.Behavioural phenotypes of hypomorphic KCC2-deficient mice. *Eur. J. Neurosci.,* 2005,21,1327-37.

Toyoda H, Ohno K, Yamada J, Ikeda M, Okabe A, Sato K, Hashimoto K, Fukuda A. Induction of NMDA and $GABA_A$ receptor-mediated $Ca^{2+}$ oscillations with KCC2 mRNA downregulation in injured facial motoneurons. *J. Neurophysiol.,* 2003, 89, 1353-1362.

Tyzio R, Minlebaev M, Rheims S, Ivanov A, Jorquera I, Holmes GL, Zilberter Y, Ben-Ari Y, Khazipov R. Postnatal changes in somatic gamma-aminobutyric acid signalling in the rat hippocampus. *Eur. J.Neurosci.,* 2008, 27, 2515-28.

Ueno T, Okabe A, Akaike N, Fukuda A, Nabekura J. Diversity of neuron-specific $K^+$-$Cl^-$ cotransporter expression and inhibitory postsynaptic potential depression in rat motoneurons. *J. Biol. Chem.,* 2002, 277, 4945-50.

Uvarov P, Ludwig A, Markkanen M, Pruunsild P, Kaila K, Delpire E, Timmusk T, Rivera C, Airaksinen MS. A novel N-terminal isoform of the neuron-specific K-Cl cotransporter KCC2. *J. Biol. Chem.,* 2007,282, 30570-6.

van den Pol AN, Obrietan K, Chen G. Excitatory actions of GABA after neuronal trauma. *J. Neurosci.,* 1996, 16, 4283-4292.

Vibat CR, Holland MJ, Kang JJ, Putney LK, O'Donnell ME. Quantitation of Na+-K+-2Cl- cotransport splice variants in human tissues using kinetic polymerase chain reaction. *Anal.Biochem.,* 2001, 298, 218-30.

Yamada J, Okabe A, Toyoda H, Kilb W, Luhmann HJ, Fukuda A. Cl- uptake promoting depolarizing GABA actions in immature rat neocortical neurons is mediated by NKCC1. *J. Physiol.,* 2004, 15, 829-41.

Yan Y, Dempsey RJ, Sun D. Expression of Na (+)-K (+)-Cl (-) cotransporter in rat brain during development and its localization in mature astrocytes. 2001, *Brain Res.,* 911, 43-55

YanY, Dempsey RJ, SunD. Na $^{+}$-K $^{+}$-Cl$^{-}$cotransporter in rat focal cerebral inchemia. *J. Cerebral. Blood Flow and Metab.,* 2001, 21, 711-721

Kanematsu T, Horibe S, Matsukawa N, Asai K, Ojika K, Hirata M, Nabekura J.Early changes in KCC2 phosphorylation in response to neuronal stress result in functional downregulation. *J. Neurosci.,* 2007, 27, 1642-1650.

Wang C, Shimizu-Okabe C, Watanabe K, Okabe A, Matsuzaki H, Ogawa T, Mori N, Fukuda A, Sato K. Developmental changes in KCC1, KCC2, and NKCC1 mRNA expressions in the rat brain. *Brain Res. Dev. Brain Res.* 2002, 139, 59-66.

Woo NS, Lu J, England R, McClellan R, Dufour S, Mount DB, Deutch AY, Lovinger DM, Delpire E. Hyperexcitability and epilepsy associated with disruption of the mouse neuronal-specific K-Clcotransporter gene. *Hippocampus,* 2002, 12, 258-268.

In: Dysplasia
Editors: L. M. Sexton and H. J. Leach
ISBN 978-1-61942-600-9


*Chapter V*

# Dysplasia in Longstanding Ulcerative Colitis: Diagnosis, Types, Surveillance and Treatment Options

***Ovidiu Fratila***
University of Oradea, Oradea, Romania

## Abstract

*Introduction:* patients with longstanding ulcerative colitis (LUC) have a high risk of developing colorectal cancer, compared to the general population. The highest risk appears in patients with extensive colitis, an intermediate risk in those having left-sided colitis whereas people with proctitis have practically no higher risk that the general population.

*Contents:* Dysplasia in UC is classified in low grade dysplasia, high grade dysplasia and indefinite for dysplasia, depending on the presence or absence of specific epithelial alterations. Protrusive lesions in UC are traditionally named DALMs (dysplasia associated lesion or mass). The degree of dysplasia is very important as it has an impact upon the sensitivity and specificity of the subsequent development of colorectal cancer. Dysplasia, irrespective of its grade, was reported to have a 74% sensitivity in the development of colorectal cancer, and in the same series studied in Mayo Clinic, high grade dysplasia had a smaller sensitivity (34%) but a 98% specificity in the detection of colorectal cancer. In a very recent meta-analysis, it was stated that the sensitivity of low grade dysplasia is associated with a 9 fold increase in the risk of developing colorectal cancer and a 12 fold increase in the risk of developing advanced neoplasia. It is therefore advisable to perform regular colonoscopic screening using different methods to detect dysplasia and/or early cancer. However this approach was not yet proved unequivocally to reduce mortality due to UC associated colorectal cancer. Beside simple colonoscopy, now there are new methods for colon surveillance: confocal chromoscopic endomicroscopy, chromoscopic colonoscopy, narrow band imaging (NBI), endoscopic trimodal imaging but these methods are not yet standardized. As treatment options, according to ECCO statements, high grade dysplasia in flat mucosa and adenocarcinoma are indications for proctocolectomy. A patient with low grade dysplasia in flat mucosa should be offered proctocolectomy or repeat surveillance biopsies within 3–6 months.

*Conclusion:* Since dysplastic changes of the colonic mucosa are associated with a high risk of colorectal cancer in patients with UC it is imperative to implement a colonoscopic surveillance program with the goal of reducing mortality and morbidity associated with colorectal cancer and in the same time to avoid unnecessary prophylactic colectomies, thus offering a less invasive treatment. Current strategies are difficult to keep, time consuming and expensive but apparently not effective enough to this purpose. Future efforts should be focused on a more accurate evaluation of individual risk factors for patient selection and an improvement of endoscopic techniques.

## INTRODUCTION

The term of ulcerative colitis belongs to Wilks și Moxon since 1875, althought Samuel Wilks makes a good description of the disease earlier, in 1859 [1].

As stated at the 2005 Montreal World Congress of Gastroenterology and later by the ECCO guidelines, ulcerative colitis is a chronic inflammatory condition causing continuous mucosal inflammation of the colon without granulomas on biopsy, affecting the rectum and a variable extent of the colon in continuity, and it is characterized by a relapsing and remitting course [2].

UC is a lifetime disease. Its etiopathology is not yet fully understood but recently, more and more evidence suggests that, similar to other inflammatory conditions, ulcerative colitis implies the immunomediated tissue disorder secondary to a variable interaction between the genetic susceptibility factors and the environmental initiating or modifying factors (figure 1). It is obvious therefore that as long as the exact etiology is not known there is no medical curative treatment yet available.

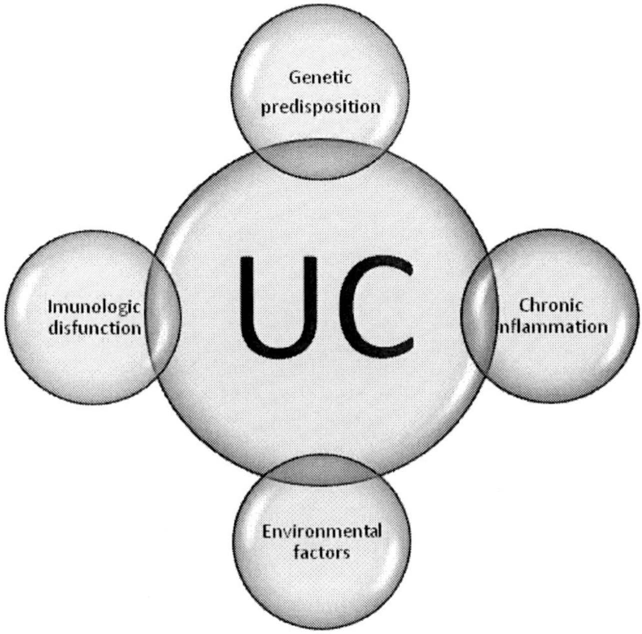


Figure 1. Sketch of the etiopathogenesis in UC.

The disease affects both men and women with a slight predominance in females. It has a bimodal age distribution, with a first major peak between 20-40 years and a second, smaller peak between 60-80 years.

The geographical distribution of UC is variable. It is more frequent in the western parts of the world than in Africa, Asia or America. In Europe there is a North-South gradient of incidence, which appears to be growing lately in south regions as well as in developing countries. Presently the disease affects almost 1 person in every 250 people from Europe and United States of America [3, 4, 5].

The prevalence of the disease is more important in people with high socio-economical levels, in those having higher work responsibility and rank, in people with high level of education, in urban areas, in white population compared with black people and in Jewish, suggesting the importance of the racial and ethnic factors [6,7].

Despite its name (ulcerative colitis), the ulceration is a late event and it is related to the severity of the disease. UC generally starts in the rectum and it either stays at this level or extends proximally. The initial lesion is poorly known. The congestive state of the mucosa with vasomotor changes and mucus over secretion demonstrates that it starts at vascular levels.

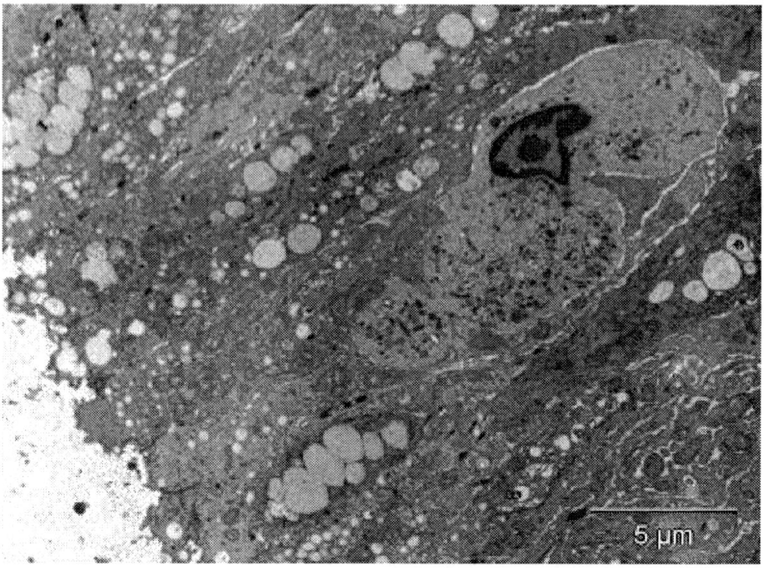


Figure 2. Neutrophil cell infiltrated through the surface epithelium cells, chorion with an altered structure, TEM (Personal collection).

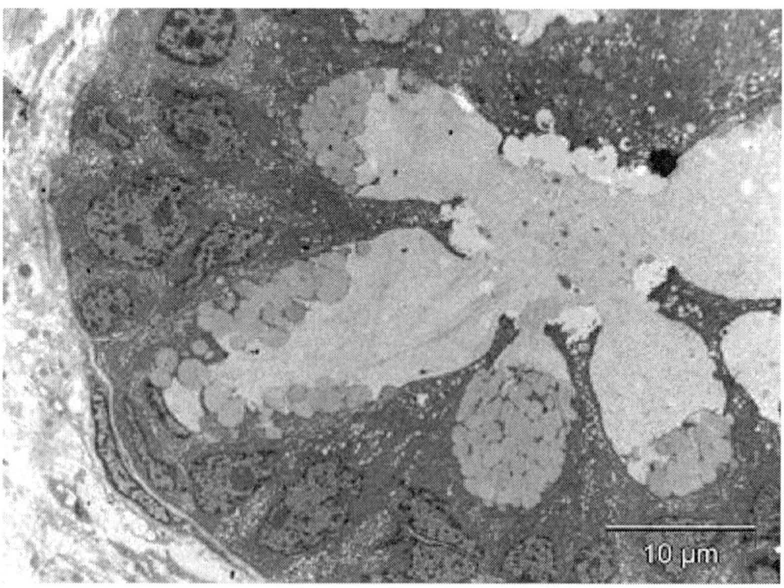


Figure 3. Gland with emptied goblet cells, TEM (personal collection).

The debut is made at the base of Lieberkuhn crypts, where the chorion gets swelled, congested and hemorrhagic suffusions are present. The mucus glands are swelled and produce important mucus secretions. The inflammatory cells infiltrate the *lamina propria* and the crypts, resulting, the well known, crypt abscesses. So, in the colon wall, diffuse inflammation of the mucosa appears, with hyperemia, granulation, pus and hemorrhagic detritus, leading in severe cases at extensive ulcerations. Later, the architecture is distorted and the goblet cells lose their mucus deposits (figure 2 and 3) [8, 9].

## Dysplasia in Ulcerative Colitis

### What Is Dysplasia?

Dysplasia is a general term for the abnormal growth or development of cells or organs. As it relates to *colon cancer,* dysplasia is the abnormal growth and development of colon cells. It is defined by the neoplastic epithelial changes capable of turning into invasive carcinoma. With referral to dysplasia, ulcerative colitis has 3 distinct categories: negative for dysplasia, indefinite for dysplasia, and positive for dysplasia. Dysplasia in then is classified into low grade dysplasia, high grade dysplasia and indefinite for dysplasia, depending on the presence or absence of specific epithelial alterations.

Protrusive lesions in UC are traditionally named DALMs (dysplasia associated lesion or mass). Dysplasia is best evaluated in areas without significant acute inflammation. However if this is not possible the diagnosis should be made positive only if the dysplastic areas are obviously disproportionate to the grade of inflammation. The final diagnosis must be confirmed by an independent pathologist according to ECCO statements.

Low grade dysplasia looks like colorectal adenomas having the same cytologic characteristics. The nuclei are enlarged and elongated and there is a frequent loss of mucin -mucus depletion (figure 4).

High grade dysplasia- a minimum of three crypts must be involved before high-grade dysplasia is diagnosed. HGD has highly atypical characteristics: pleomorphic cells, important cytological atypia, nuclear stratification extended to the surface of the epithelial cells with loss of polarity (figure 5).

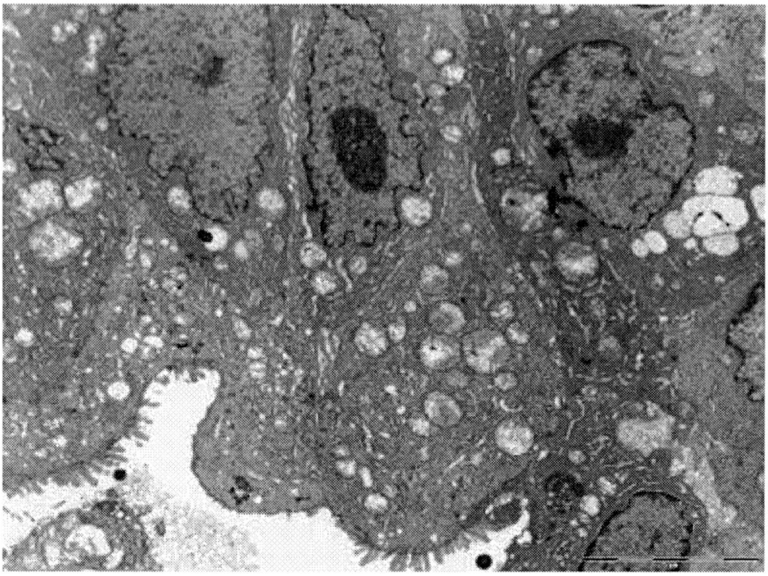

Figure 4. Transitional mucosa, TEM (personal collection).

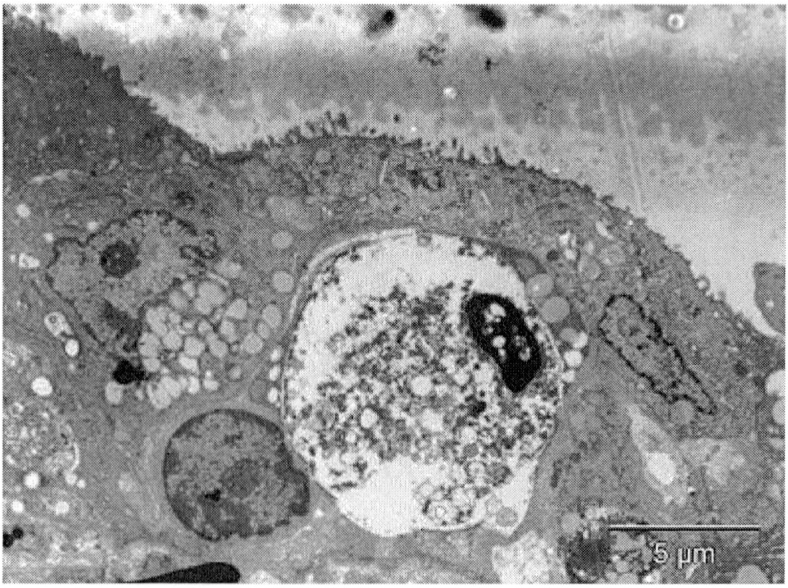


Figure 5. High grade dysplasia, TEM (personal collection).

Indefinite for dysplasia cases are difficult to diagnose and it means that although there are some epithelial changes suggestive for dysplasia they are not defiantly diagnostic of dysplasia. It is often used when the intense active inflammation is blurring the interpretation [10]. Cancer development is more frequent in chronically active forms of UC rather than in recurrent forms and also in cases with coexistent sclerosing colangitis, family history of colorectal cancer, adenomatous polyps on the affected mucosa, folat deficiency and lack of 5-ASA treatment [11].

## Why Looking for Dysplasia in UC?

***Because of the Risk of Developing Colonic Cancer!***

Patients with longstanding ulcerative colitis (LUC) have a high risk of developing colorectal cancer, compared to the general population, through a chronic inflammation- dysplasia -carcinoma sequence (figure 6).

The highest risk appears in patients with extensive colitis, an intermediate risk in those having left-sided colitis whereas people with proctitis have practically no higher risk that the general population.

The risk of developing colorectal cancer is increased in patients with duration of at least 7-10 years and having total and subtotal colitis. The risk rate differs between certain populations and certain studies that are taken into account, malignant tumors rising in UC patients having a 7-30 fold increase than the general population. The cumulative risk of developing cancer after 30 years of disease is 20% [12, 13, 14,15].

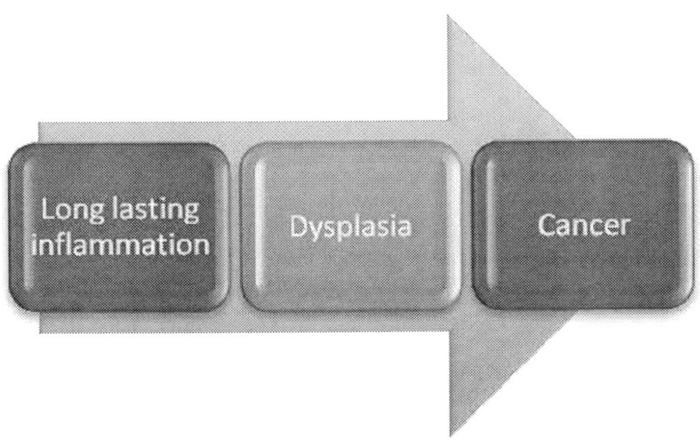


Figure 6. Sequence of the development of carcinoma.

The grade of dysplasia is very important as it has an impact upon the sensibility and the specificity of the presence and future development of colorectal cancer [16].

Dysplasia, irrespective of its grade, was reported to have 74% sensitivity in the development of colorectal cancer, and in the same series studied in Mayo Clinic, high grade dysplasia had a smaller sensitivity (34%) but 98% specificity in the detection of colorectal cancer [17].

In a very recent meta-analysis, it was stated that the sensitivity of low grade dysplasia is associated with a 9 fold increase in the risk of developing colorectal cancer and a 12 fold increase in the risk of developing advanced neoplasia [18].

Microscopically UC associated cancer is usually an adenocarcinoma and occasionally it has a high production of mucus.

### *So, Who Should We Screen?*

According to several well documented studies it is compulsory to screen all patients with ulcerative colitis that have longstanding disease, extensive forms, and sclerosing colangitis [19, 20, 21]. There are some situations in which screening is still recommended but the evidence are not so well established and these categories are: early (<20 yrs) onset of disease, family history of colorectal cancer, persistent activity of the disease [22, 23,24].

In extensive colitis patients, the screening colonoscopy should be performed every 2 years until 20 years of disease and afterwards it should be done once a year. In distal or left side colitis cases the surveillance should start after 15 years of the disease and in patients with proctitis this kind of surveillance is not necessary [25]. If biopsies are indefinite for dysplasia (confirmed by an experimented anatomopathologist) it is advisable to perform colonoscopy at a 3-6 month interval, with a concomitant increase of the treatment [26, 27].

### *How Should We Diagnose and Screen?*

As it is well known, colonoscopy represents the preferred way to perform colorectal cancer surveillance in patients with UC.

At the beginning of the colonoscopic surveillance program an initial colonoscopy is performed in order to revaluate the extent of the disease and to confirm the absence of dysplastic changes.

The final goal of the surveillance colonoscopy is to identify if the colonic mucosa has started to make the first step towards malignant transformation, so to detect dysplasia and therefore identifying the UC patients most likely to develop colorectal cancer.

The moment UC becomes longstanding (after 7-10 years of evolution), colonoscopy is recommended once or twice a year with multiple biopsies.

There are still differences in expert opinions whether to collect multiple biopsies every 10 cm (ACG) or to collect random biopsies (one biopsy from each of the four quadrants, every 10 cm) and targeted biopsies of any visible lesion should be performed during surveillance colonoscopy (ECCO).

Many researchers demonstrated that usually most dysplasia cases are recognizable during colonoscopy. As much as ¾ of the cases of definite dysplasia had a previously described abnormality obtained by the endoscopist during the procedure [28, 29, 30].

Dysplasia might arise focally thus adequate sampling is compulsory.

According to the studies of Rubin et al the number of biopsies needed to obtain a 90% sensitivity is 33 [31]. Surveillance colonoscopic programs are widely used but unfortunately they didn't manage to decrease mortality due to UC associated colorectal cancer. It is therefore obvious the need to increase the accuracy and precocity of the diagnosis of dysplasia in UC [32, 33, 34, 35, 36, 37].

### *New Methods for Colon Surveillance*

There are some novel endoscopic techniques that aim to detect with a higher accuracy the problematic areas in UC mucosa such as minimally raised lesions or flat lesions.

These are:

*Contrast enhanced endoscopy- chromo and optical contrast techniques:*

- *Chromoendoscopy* (dye staining- metilen blue) = Chromoscopic colonoscopy
- Narrow Band Imaging (NBI) -optical contrast technique
- MBI (computed virtual chromoendoscopy system) and iScan-dependent on computed spectral estimation technology) same principle like NBI but they are not dependent on optical filters.
- Fluorescence imaging (AFI)– auto fluorescence technique

- Confocal laser endomicroscopy – high resolution imaging of cellular and subcellular tissue when optical slices of mucosal surface created by detecting reflected light and tissue autofluorescence enhances through the administration of fluorescent contrast agent
- Endoscopic trimodal imaging (ETMI) incorporates high resolution endoscopy (HRE), autofluorescence imaging (AFI) and narrow band imaging (NBI)
- Molecular imaging - in vivo molecular imaging with fluorescent leveling of cells by their molecular features - has been recently introduced and it represents the true development in contrast enhanced endoscopic technologies [38].

Studies that used these methods either alone or in comparison with white light colonoscopy reported better detection rates of dysplasia, varying from a 1,5 to 5 times increase in accuracy [39, 40,41,42, 43, 44, 45 ].

At present, none of these methods are widely recommended for routine screening of patients with longstanding UC but rather for those patients known to have low grade dysplasia or indefinite for dysplasia cases (without colectomy) and in need to close follow up.

## *Once Found, What to Do With It?*

### Treatment

First of all, because of the large intraobserver variability, dysplastic changes must be confirmed by a second independent, experienced pathologist, preferably with a dedicated work to the gastrointestinal tract. HGD in flat mucosa and adenocarcinoma are indications for proctocolectomy. Patients that have LGD must be offered either the choice of a proctocolectomy or an intensive surveillance program with repeated biopsies at 3-6 month intervals [46]. Taking into account that some prospective studies with UC and LGD, showed a low rate of developing colorectal cancer, some experts consider reasonable the compromise of continuing the biopsy ingathering at these short intervals but only for those patients that are willing to strictly adhere to this surveillance program [47, 48]. Protrusive lesions, traditionally named DALM-s (dysplasia associated lesion or mass) had until recently an absolute indication for colectomy. But it was later observed that some of these lesions might be like sporadic adenomas so they can be successfully treated by complete endoscopic resection. [49, 50]. If complete polipectomy is then confirmed by histology and if the biopsies obtained by the adjacent flat mucosa are free of dysplastic changes, and moreover if there are no other dysplastic areas thought the colon then the colectomy might be safely postponed. Further colonoscopic surveillance (3-6 month intervals) is necessary as some of these patients might develop other protrusive lesions. If these new lesions do not resemble typical adenomas or if the surrounding mucosa has dysplastic changes then colectomy is the right choice because of the risk of CRC development.

The prognostic of the patients with CRC and UC is the same like in those without UC and unequivocal evidence that surveillance colonoscopy prolongs survival in patients with UC is lacking [46].

## CONCLUSION

Since dysplastic changes of the colonic mucosa are associated with a high risk of colorectal cancer in patients with UC it is imperative to widely use and implement a colonoscopic surveillance program with the goal of reducing mortality and morbidity associated with colorectal cancer and in the same time to avoid unnecessary prophylactic colectomies, thus offering a less invasive treatment. Current strategies are difficult to keep, time consuming and expensive but apparently not effective enough to this purpose. Future efforts should be focused on a more accurate evaluation of individual risk factors for patient selection and an improvement of endoscopic techniques.

## REFERENCES

[1] *Wilks S*, Moxon W. *Lectures on Pathological anatomy* 2 no edn. London, Brown Green, Longmans Roberts and Co., 1875; 465-466.

[2] Silverberg MS, Satsangi J, Ahmad T, et al. Toward an integrated clinical,molecular and serological classification of inflammatory bowel disease: report of a working party of the 2005 Montreal World Congress of Gastroenterology. *Can. J. Gastroenterol* 2005;19(Suppl A):5–36.

[3] S Shivananda, J Lennard-Jones, R Logan, N Fear, A Price, L Carpenter, M van Blankenstein Incidence of inflammatory bowel disease across Europe: is there a difference between north and south? *Results of the European Collaborative Study on Inflammatory Bowel Disease (EC-IBD).* Gut 1996;39:690-697.

[4] Lakatos, Peter Laszlo Recent trends in the epidemiology of inflammatory boweldiseases: Up or down? *World J. Gastroenterol* 2006 October 14; 12(38): 6102-6108.

[5] Ghosh S, Mitchell R. Impact of inflammatory bowel disease on quality of life: Results of the European Federation of Crohn's and Ulcerative colitis Associations (EFFCA) patient survey. *J. Crohn's Colitis* 2007;1:10-20.

[6] Bernstein CN, Blanchard JF, Rawsthorne P, Wajda A. Epidemiology of Crohn's disease and ulcerative colitis in a central Canadian province: a population-based study. *Am. J. Epidemiol.* 1999 May 15;149(10):916-24.

[7] Farmer RG, Easley KA, Rankin GB.Clinical patterns, natural history, and progression of ulcerative colitis. A long-term follow-up of 1116 patients. *Dig. Dis. Sci.* 1993 Jun;38(6):1137-46.

[8] Schumacher G, Sandstedt B, Kollberg B. A prospective study of first attacks of inflammatory bowel disease and infectious colitis. Clinical findings and early diagnosis. *Scand. J. Gastroenterol.* 1994 Mar;29(3):265-74.

[9] C A Seldenrijk, B C Morson, S G Meuwissen, Histopathological evaluation of colonic mucosal biopsy specimens in chronic inflammatory bowel disease: *diagnostic implications*. Gut 1991; 32: 1514-1520.

[10] Riddell RH, Goldman H, Ransohoff DF, et al. Dysplasia in inflammatory bowel disease: standardized classification with provisional clinical applications. *Hum. Pathol.* 1983;14(11):931-968.

[11] Salmo Emil , Patrick O'Connolly and Najib Haboubi, Dysplasia in Inflammatory Bowel Disease: from Genetics to Treatment, *Inflammatory Bowel Disease and Familial Adenomatous Polyposis ,* Section II, 35-44, 2006.

[12] Bernstein CN, Blanchard JF, Kliewer E, Wajda A. Cancer risk in patients with inflammatory bowel disease: a population-based study. *Cancer.* 2001 Feb 15;91(4):854-62.

[13] Ekbom Anders , Risk of cancer in ulcerative colitis, *Journal of Gastrointestinal Surgery,* Volume 2, Number 4, 312-313.

[14] Eaden JA, Abrams KR, Mayberry JF. *The risk of colorectal cancer in ulcerative colitis: a meta-analysis.* Gut. 2001 Apr;48(4):526-35.

[15] Stewénius J. , I. Adnerhill, H. Anderson, G. R. Ekelund, C. -H. Florén, F. -T. Fork, L. Janzon, C. Lindström and M. Ögren Incidence of colorectal cancer and all cause mortality in non-selected patients with

ulcerative colitis and indeterminate colitis in Malmö, Sweden, *International Journal of Colorectal Disease Volume* 10, , 1995, Number 2, 117-122.

[16] Taylor BA, Pemberton JH, Carpenter HA, Levin KE, Schroeder KW, Welling DR, Spencer MP, Zinsmeister AR. Dysplasia in chronic ulcerative colitis: implications for colonoscopic surveillance. *Dis. Colon. Rectum.* 1992 Oct;35(10):950-6.

[17] Suhal S. Mahid, et al, Smoking and Inflammatory Bowel Disease: A Meta-analysis, Mayo Clinic Proceedings November 2006 vol. 81 no. 11 1462-147.

[18] Thomas T, Abrams KA, Robinson RJ, Mayberry JF. Meta-analysis: cancer risk of low-grade dysplasia in chronic ulcerative colitis. *Aliment Pharmacol Ther.* 2007 Mar 15;25(6):657-68.

[19] Colon cancer: *The risk of colorectal cancer in ulcerative colitis: a meta-analysis* J A Eaden, K R Abrams, J F MayberryGut 2001;48:526-535.

[20] Increased risk of colorectal neoplasia in patients with primary sclerosing cholangitis and ulcerative colitis: a meta-analysis. Soetikno RM, Lin OS, Heidenreich PA, Young HS, Blackstone MO *Gastrointest Endosc.* 2002;56(1):48-54.

[21] Collins P, Rhodes J. Ulcerative colitis: diagnosis and management. *BMJ.* 2006; 333:340-343.

[22] Colon cancer: *The risk of colorectal cancer in ulcerative colitis: a meta-analysis* J A Eaden, K R Abrams, J F MayberryGut 2001;48:526-535.

[23] Nuako KW, Ahlquist DA, Mahoney DW, Schaid DJ, Siems DM, Lindor NM. Gastroenterology. Familial predisposition for colorectal cancer in chronic ulcerative colitis: *a case-control study,* 1998 Nov;115(5):1079-83.

[24] Rutter M, Saunders B, Wilkinson K, et al. Severity of inflammation is a risk factor of colorectal neoplasia in ulcerative colitis. *Gastroenterology* 2004;126:451-9.

[25] Itzkowitz SH, Present DH; Crohn's and Colitis Foundation of America Colon Cancer in IBD Study Group. Consensus conference: Colorectal cancer screening and surveillance in inflammatory bowel disease. *Inflamm. Bowel Dis.* 2005 Mar;11(3):314-21.

[26] Chambers WM, Warren BF, Jewell DP, Mortensen NJ. Cancer surveillance in ulcerative colitis. *Br. J. Surg.* 2005 Aug;92(8):928-36.

[27] Obrador A, Ginard D, Barranco L. Review article: colorectal cancer surveillance in ulcerative colitis - what should we be doing? *Aliment Pharmacol Ther.* 2006 Oct;24 Suppl 3:56-63.

[28] Rutter MD , Saunders BP , Wilkinson KH et al. Most dysplasia in ulcerative colitis is visible at colonoscopy . *Gastrointest. Endosc.* 2004 ; 60 : 334 – 9 .

[29] Rubin DT , Rothe JA , Hetzel JT e t al. Are dysplasia and colorectal cancer endoscopically visible in patients with ulcerative colitis? *Gastrointest. Endosc.* 2007 ; 65 : 998 – 1004 .

[30] Blonski W , Kundu R , Lewis J et al. Is dysplasia visible during surveillance colonoscopy in patients with ulcerative colitis? *Scand. J. Gastroenterol* 2008 ; 43 : 698 – 703 .

[31] Rubin CE, Haggitt RC, Burmer GC, Brentnall TA, Stevens AC, Levine DS, Dean PJ, Kimmey M, Perera DR, Rabinovitch PS DNA aneuploidy in colonic biopsies predicts future development of dysplasia in ulcerative colitis. *Gastroenterology* 1992, 103(5):1611-20.

[32] Charles N. Bernstein Neoplasia in inflammatory bowel disease: Surveillance and management strategies Current *Gastroenterology Reports* Volume 8, Number 6, 513-518.

[33] Charles N. Bernstein, How do we assess the value of surveillance techniques in ulcerative colitis? *Journal of Gastrointestinal Surgery,* Volume 2, Number 4, 318-321.

[34] Iris Dotan, Inflammatory bowel disease and colorectal cancer: What is new? *Current Colorectal Cancer Reports,*Volume 5, Number 1, 35-39.

[35] Mitchell P. J., E. Salmo and N. Y. Haboubi Inflammatory bowel disease: the problems of dysplasia and surveillance Case Report, *Techniques in Coloproctology* Volume 11, Number 4, 299-309.

[36] Svrcek Magali and J. F. Fléjou, Aspects anatomopathologiques des lésions précancéreuses survenant dans le cadre des maladies inflammatoires chroniques de l'intestin (MICI), *Acta. Endoscopica* Volume 36, Number 5, 689-700.

[37] Catherine, Rodger Haggitt and Robert Riddell Dysplasia in inflammatory bowel disease: clinical pathology and current surveillance methods, Inflammatory *Bowel Disease: From Bench to Bedside,* Section II, 719-729, 2005.

[38] Successful training in gastrointestinal endoscopy, First edition, edited by Jonathan Cohen, *Blackwell Publishing* ltd pg 159-169, 2011.

[39] Kiesslich R, Galle PR , Neurath MF . Endoscopic surveillance in ulcerative colitis: smart biopsies do it better. *Gastroenterology* 2007, 133 : 742 – 5.

[40] Kiesslich R, Goetz M, Lammersdorf K e t al. Chromoscopy-guided endomicroscopy increases the diagnostic yield of intraepithelial neoplasia in ulcerative colitis . *Gastroenterology* 2007 ; 132 : 874 – 82 .

[41] Hurlstone DP, McAlindon ME , Sanders DS e t al. Further validation of high-magnifi cation chromoscopic-colonoscopy for the detection of intraepithelial neoplasia and colon cancer in ulcerative colitis . *Gastroenterology* 2004; 126 : 376 – 8 .

[42] Hurlstone DP , Sanders DS , Lobo AJ e t al. Indigo carmine-assisted highmagnification chromoscopic colonoscopy for the detection and characterization of intraepithelial neoplasia in ulcerative colitis: a prospective evaluation. *Endoscopy* 2005 ; 37 : 1186 – 92 .

[43] Kiesslich R , Fritsch J , Holtmann M e t al. Methylene blue-aided chromoendoscopy for the detection of intraepithelial neoplasia and colon cancer in ulcerative colitis . *Gastroenterology* 2003 ; 124 : 880 – 8.

[44] Rutter MD , Saunders BP , Schofi eld G et al. *Pancolonic indigo carmine dye spraying for the detection of dysplasia in ulcerative colitis* . Gut 2004 ; 53 : 256 – 60.

[45] Marion JF , Waye JD , Present DH et al. Chromoendoscopy-targeted biopsies are superior to standard colonoscopic surveillance for detecting dysplasia in infl ammatory bowel disease patients: a prospective endoscopic trial . *Am. J .Gastroenterol* 2008 ; 103 : 2342 – 9.

[46] Livia Biancone, Pierre Michetti, Simon Travis, Johanna C. Escher, Gabriele Moser, Alastair Forbes, Jörg C Hoffmann, Axel Dignass, Paolo Gionchetti, Günter Jantschek, Ralf Kiesslich, Sanja Kolacek, Rod Mitchell, Julian Panes, Johan Soderholm, Boris Vucelic, Eduard Stang, for the European Crohn's and Colitis Organisation (ECCO), European evidence-based Consensus on the management of ulcerative colitis: *Special situations Journal of Crohn's and Colitis* (2008) 2, 63–92.

[47] Befrits R, Ljung T, Jaramillo E, Rubio C. Low-grade dysplasia in extensive, long-standing inflammatory bowel disease: a follow-up study. *Dis. Colon. Rectum.* 2002 May;45(5):615-20.

[48] Collins PD, Mpofu C, Watson AJ, Rhodes JM. Strategies for detecting colon cancer and/or dysplasia in patients with inflammatory bowel disease. *Cochrane Database of Systematic Reviews* 2006.

[49] Engelsgjerd M, Farraye FA, Odze RD. Polypectomy may be adequate treatment for adenoma-like dysplastic lesions in chronic ulcerative colitis. *Gastroenterology.* 1999 Dec;117(6):1288-94; discussion 1488-91.

[50] Peter H. Rubin, Sonya Friedman, Noam Harpaz, Eric Goldstein, Jeffrey Weiser, Jeremy Schiller, Jerome D. Waye, Daniel H. Present Colonoscopic polypectomy in chronic colitis: Conservative management after endoscopic resection of dysplastic polyps *Gastroenterology* 1 December 1999, volume 117 issue 6 Pages 1295-1300.

In: Dysplasia
Editors: L. M. Sexton and H. J. Leach
ISBN 978-1-61942-600-9


*Chapter VI*

# CHARACTERIZATION OF ANGIOGENIC ACTIVITY AND IDENTIFICATION OF MEDIATORS IN BRONCHIAL DYSPLASIA AND INVASIVE LUNG CANCER: ROLE OF VASCULAR ENDOTHELIAL GROWTH FACTOR AND ANGIOPOIETINS

***D. T. Merrick[1,2], S. Petrunich[1,2], Y. E. Miller[1,2], R. L. Keith, T. C. Kennedy[1] and W. A. Franklin[1]***

[1] Departments of Pathology and Medicine/Pulmonary, University of Colorado Cancer Center, US

[2] Departments of Pathology and Medicine/Pulmonary, Denver Veteran's Administration Medical Center, Denver, Colorado, US

## ABSTRACT

*Introduction:* Bronchial dysplasia is the most common premalignant lesion found in lung. In addition to other alterations, we have previously shown that in comparison to normal bronchial mucosa, bronchial dysplasia demonstrates increased vascular endothelial growth factor (VEGF) expression and increased angiogenic activity as measured by microvessel densities. The characterization of angiogenesis in bronchial dysplasia has been extended herein to include analysis of other angiogenic factors and to establish a mechanistic relationship between factor expression and angiogenic activity.

*Materials and Methods: In situ* characterization of angiogenic factor expression has been performed via quantitative RT-PCR on frozen tissue from 64 bronchial biopsies and 34 matched tumor-normal pairs. Epithelial cultures from bronchial biopsies representing a range of histologies have been used to study effects of conditioned media on endothelial cell proliferation, migration and tubulogenesis.

*Results:* Characterization of angiopoietin pathway factor expression shows that levels of angiopoietin-1, angiopoietin-2 and their receptor Tie2 are not different between bronchial dysplasia and normal bronchial epithelium, but are reduced in tumor tissue as compared to its matched normal tissue. Conditioned media from cultures of bronchial dysplasia shows induction of endothelial cell proliferation (5/6 dysplasia cell lines), migration (6/7) and tubule elongation (5/6) but no induction of new tubule formation (0/6). Addition of neutralizing anti-VEGF antibody completely abrogates proliferation, migration and tubule elongation induced by dysplasia derived conditioned media in nearly all cell lines tested.

*Conclusions:* Angiogenic activity in bronchial dysplasia appears to be largely mediated by VEGF. Although other factors may contribute to angiogenesis in bronchial dysplasia in some cases, this appears to be more prominent in invasive lung cancer. Features that distinguish angiogenic activity in bronchial dysplasia versus invasive lung cancer will be discussed. The potential interaction between angiopoietin and VEGF mediated angiogenesis in the development of lung cancer is explored. Distinct characteristics of bronchial dysplasia associated angiogenesis may have important implications in using these factors as markers of bronchial dysplasia or as targets for chemoprevention in lung cancer.

## INTRODUCTION

Angiogenesis refers to the recruitment of vasculature to provide additional nutrients for tissue in which there is increased metabolic demand. This activity has been documented by a variety of methods in a number of pathologic processes including tissue repair, reactive proliferation and neoplasia. It has been demonstrated to be essential for the growth of tumors and data suggest that without the recruitment of new vessels, neoplastic lesions cannot grow beyond .4 mm in diameter [1]. A large number of angiogenic factors have been described and induction of angiogenic activity is controlled by a delicate balance between pro- and anti-angiogenic factors in tissue. Angiogenic factors orchestrate a variety of different affects on vascular structures. Angiogenic activity is characterized by extension of vasculature structures and proliferation of the cellular constituents of vessels. The stimulation of endothelial cell and pericyte proliferation and migration are primary activities mediated by angiogenic factors. Vessel growth is accompanied by varying degrees of branching or capillary budding and lumen formation (tubulogenesis). In addition, vascular maturational processes such as mural smooth muscle recruitment and stabilization and vessel functionality can be altered by regulating vessel wall integrity and vascular permeability. Each angiogenic factor acts as a primary inducer or inhibitor of one or more of these activities, and the nature of angiogenesis may emphasize some of these activities over others depending on the type of process or stage of the disease in which the angiogenic activity is taking place. Given these varied activities, it can be suggested that angiogenic activity generally fits into two overlapping but distinct categories. The stimulation of endothelial cell proliferation and migration can be considered the primary features of the “proliferative phase” of angiogenesis whereas mural wall constituent establishment, regulation of permeability and terminal capillary sprouting are characteristic of the “maturational phase.”

Vascular endothelial growth factor (VEGF) is the most potent inducer of endothelial cell proliferation and migration to have been described [1], although fibroblast growth factor (FGF) is also known to strongly promote these activities. VEGF can also induce vascular maturation and mediate alterations in vascular permeability. While platelet derived growth factor (PDGF) can have some effect on these processes, it appears to primarily contribute to maturational activities by inducing pericyte proliferation and migration. For each of these angiogenic factors there are a set of transmembrane receptors with which they interact to mediate their angiogenic affects. The type of activity that is induced is determined to a great degree by which receptor the ligand interacts with and by features of the cell in which that interaction is occurring. VEGF is secreted by a variety of cell types including epithelial cells, but the expression of its receptors (VEGFRs) is generally restricted to endothelial cells. When binding to VEGFR2 (also known as KDR) is the primary receptor interaction, VEGF will generally induce endothelial cell proliferation and migration [2]. However, when VEGFR1 (also known as flt-1) is present in significant amounts, proliferative activity is not prominent and endothelial effects of VEGF appear to be diverted to maturational or differentiation related activities and regulation of vascular permeability [3,4]. Heterodimerization between VEGFR1 and 2 alters downstream signaling within endothelial cells such that it is primarily mediated through the phospholipase-Cγ1 (PLCγ1) rather than the phosphoinositol-3-kinase (PI3K) pathway and it is thought that this is central to determining the ultimate cellular effect of VEGF activity [5-7]. Alternatively VEGFR2 homodimerazation or heterodimerization with an additional VEGF receptor, neuropilin-1 (nrp-1) stimulates PI3K activity and therefore appears to lead primarily to proliferative activity. An additional level of complexity is added to VEGF signaling via the existence of multiple isoforms of the VEGF ligand. These ligands have restricted activity by virtue of differences in the receptors with which they interact and their bioavailability. VEGF121 acts as a ligand for VEGFR2 almost exclusively, while VEGF165 can interact with VEGFR1, VEGFR2 and nrp-1. Larger isoforms (189, 205, etc.) are sequestered in the extracellular matrix by interactions with heparan sulfates and thus mediate effects on vascular permeability only when released from the extracellular matrix in inflammatory or other processes [8]. Table 1 summarizes the varied actions associated with VEGF mediated angiogenic activity and gives a general outline of the specific ligand isoforms and receptors involved in directing VEGF activity.

There is significant overlap in these activites and the categorization presented in this table should be considered a simplified representation. Angiopoietins, angiostatins and other factors are generally regarded as mediators of vascular maturation and either inhibit angiogenic proliferative activities or divert angiogenic activity toward differentiation associated processes. Angiopoietin activity is mediated by four ligands which interact with a single receptor, Tie2, that is expressed on endothelium and vessel associated smooth muscle cells and pericytes [9-12]. Angiopoietin 1 (Ang1) is the main Tie2 ligand and the prototypical Tie2 agonist [13,14]. Conversely, angiopoietin 2 (Ang2) is an antagonist ligand for Tie2 [15]. Ang1 induces endothelial cell migration, tubulogenesis and sprouting but not endothelial cell proliferation [13,16,17 23,24 in angp1]. Some of these activities, especially induction of new vascular sprouts, are suspected to be mediated via cooperative activity involving VEGF [18]. However, the primary role of Ang1 in promoting vessel maturation has been further supported by observations demonstrating Ang1 induction of smooth muscle precursor cell migration and maintenance of mature vascular smooth muscle in angiogenesis models [10,12]. In the lack of such maturation associated mural investiture, vessels generally demonstrate high proliferative activity and permeability, characteristics changes seen in tumor vasculature. Indeed, xenograft models have demonstrated inhibition of tumor and premalignant lesion growth by ectopic expression of Ang1 [19]. On the other hand, Ang2 appears to antagonize maturational activities such as mural cell recruitment [15]. If expressed in the presence of VEGF, Ang2 has been shown to induce endothelial cell proliferation and migration as well vessel sprouting [20]. These features of angiopoetin activity have led to a model in which tumor angiogenesis would be supposed to demonstrate preferential Ang2 expression in comparison to Ang1 expression. However, studies of a number of tumors have produced conflicting data regarding this expression profile. In lung cancer, previous publications have detected consistent overexpression of Ang2 in comparison to normal tissue but have variably demonstrated increased or decreased Ang1 expression [21, 22].

**Table 1. Table showing characteristics of VEGF isoforms and receptors and summarizing the activities associated with these mediators of VEGF activity**

| | Receptor Interactions | | | Endothelial cell actions | | | ECM interactions | |
|---|---|---|---|---|---|---|---|---|
| | VEGFR-1 | VEGFR-2 | NRP-1 | Prolif & Migration | Migration& Tubulogen. | Perm. & Vasodil. | Interact | %Bound |
| VEGF121 | +/- | + | - | ++ | -** | ++ | - | 0 |
| VEGF145 | - | + | - | + | + | | + | High |
| VEGF165 | + | + | + | +++ | + | ++ | + | 70 |
| VEGF189 (+183) | -* | -* | -* | -* | ++ | - | + | 100 |
| VEGF206 | -* | -* | -* | -* | | | + | 100 |

* VEGF183/189/206 can be associated with low levels of VEGFR binding and endothelial cell proliferation after proteolytic activiation by plasmin.

** *In vitro* assays show positive effect of VEGF121 on EDC adhesion and migration, but *in vivo* observations suggest it mediates intralumenal EDC proliferation without new vessel formation.

The role of angiogenesis in cancer propagation and metastatic activity has been extensively studied. Numerous studies have associated angiogenic activity or expression of angiogenic factors with prognosis in esophagus, breast, head and neck and several other types of cancer [23-25]. In NSCLC increased expression of VEGF has been demonstrated in a number of publications and this overexpression has been correlated with poor prognosis or tumor stage in several of these works [26, 27]. In addition, some have found an association between increased expression of specific VEGF isoforms or VEGFR2 expression and prognosis in non-small cell lung carcinoma (NSCLC) [26,28]. While some of these publications have correlated VEGF levels with MVD suggesting a mechanistic link between VEGF expression and angiogenesis, our data did not show a statistically significant correlation between these measurements suggesting that overall angiogenic activity may be influenced by other angiogenic factors in both early preinvasive and invasive lung cancer [26,29,30]. Indeed, increased expression of pro-angiogenic factors such as hepatocyte growth factor (HGF), platelet derived – endothelial cell growth factor (PD-ECGF), basic fibroblast growth factor (bFGF/FGF2), the family of ELR containing CXC chemokines and angiopoietins have all been reported in lung cancer [rev. in 31] In addition, increased HGF and FGF2 are associated with poor prognosis, and ELR-CXC chemokines, PD-ECGF and FGF2 have been associated with increased levels of angiogenesis as measured by MVD or similar assays. In respect to VEGF expression, our previous work has also demonstrated distinctive patterns of VEGF isoform and receptor expression in bronchial dysplasia, stage I and stage II/III invasive NSCLC suggesting that the general character of VEGF mediated angiogenesis is different at the various stages of lung cancer development [32]. Finally, no studies have to this point demonstrated a mechanistic link between VEGF expression in bronchial dysplasia or invasive lung cancer and angiogenic activity. Thus, in order to fully understand angiogenic activity in the development of lung cancer, we must more closely study the interactions between angiogenic factors and also develop assays to characterize the actual mechanistic effects of the angiogenic factors elaborated by bronchial dysplasias and lung cancers.

The importance of acquiring angiogenic activity in pre-invasive dysplastic lesions has not been well established, however a growing volume of evidence supporting the frequent presence of angiogenic change in premalignant lesions in many types of tissue suggests that this is a common and likely important feature in the development and progression of premalignancy. This may be particularly prominent in lung, where a histologically distinctive lesion showing papillary tufts of capillary structures extending into overlying dysplastic epithelium has been described and given the specific classification of angiogenic squamous dysplasia (ASD) [33]. Our work has established that VEGF expression is increased in bronchial dysplasias, including ASD, and has shown that these lesions may have distinct profiles in respect to the angiogenic factors when compared to normal/reactive tissue and invasive carcinomas. In order to understand the importance of angiogenesis in bronchial dysplasia we have conducted analyses designed to determine what other angiogenic factors may be contributing to this activity and have employed *in vitro* analyses of dysplasia associated stimulation of endothelial cell activities to help define the mechanistic role of VEGF in producing these actions. Characterizing these features of dysplasia associated angiogenesis will allow for more informed decisions regarding the identification of targets for potentially effective anti-angiogenic chemopreventive therapies in this disease and point to the most informative markers of this process in bronchial dysplasia. The implications of the results presented herein are discussed in respect to their importance in characterizing premalignant change in the bronchial tree and possible implications regarding the natural history of dysplastic lesions.

# MATERIALS AND METHODS

## Subjects and Specimens

RNA from bronchial biopsy derived tissue was used for previously assayed expression levels of VEGF [32] and for newly assayed expression levels of the angiopoietins Ang1 and Ang2 and their receptor Tie2. Bronchial biopsies were collected from high-risk smoker subjects recruited to two Colorado SPORE in lung cancer trials, one composed of patients without known lung cancer and the other composed of patients with concurrent lung carcinoma. The biopsies were obtained using fluorescent bronchoscopy and subjects were enrolled using the following high risk criteria: 1) greater than 30 pack year smoking histories, 2) clinically documented pulmonary function indicating airway obstruction and 3) cytologic atypia on sputum analysis. In addition, a few normal specimens came from normal never smoker volunteers recruited as control subjects for these bronchoscopy trials. Sixty-two biopsies were analyzed including 15 normal (3 from never smokers), four reserve cell hyperplasias, 19 low grade (mild) dysplasias and 24 high grade (moderate, severe and carcinoma-in-situ) dysplasias (figure 1). These biopsies were classified according to WHO/IASLC approved criterion. RNA was collected from biopsies that were flash frozen in liquid nitrogen immediately after collection and then subsequently processed by frozen section in a -28°C crytome. Sections for hematoxylin and eosin stained slides were obtained at superficial, mid and deep levels to document histologic characteristics for each specimen. The intervening sections were transferred to Trizol reagent (GibcoBRL, Grand Island, New York) with care not to allow thawing of the tissue before placement in the RNA extraction solution. One milliliter aliquots of Trizol were extracted with 200 μl of chloroform followed by removal of the aqueous phase and precipitation with 500 μl of isopropanol at -70°C for one hour. The RNA precipitate was washed with 200 μl of 70% ethanol and resuspended in 500 μl of DEPC water. RNA concentration was determined for each specimen by measuring absorbance at 260 nm. RNA integrity was analyzed for several specimens utilizing an actin based duplex PCR assay that compares relative levels of immediate 5' and mid cDNA products [34]. Nearly all of the bronchial biopsy derived RNA tested demonstrated PCR product ratios indicating high quality by this assay.

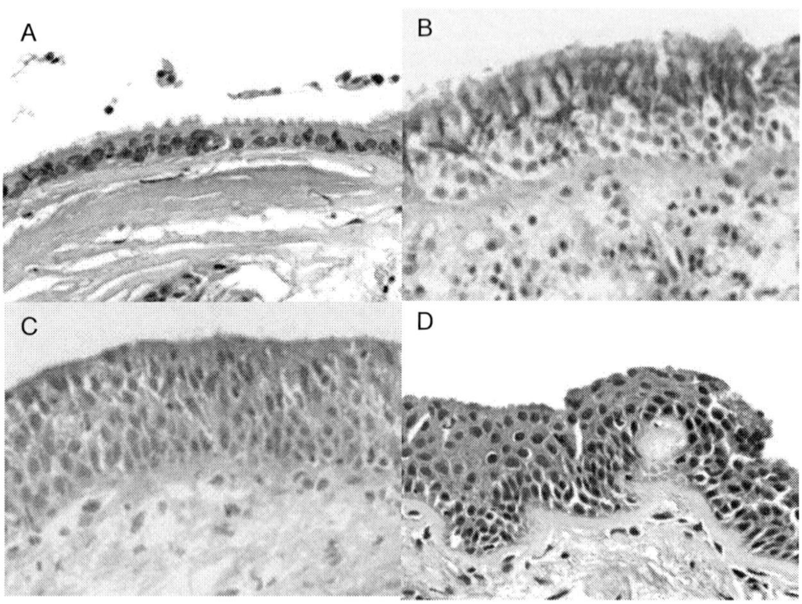


Figure 1. Hematoxylin and Eosin stained sections of bronchial epithelium representing normal (A), reserve cell hyperplasia (B), low-grade dysplasia (C) and high-grade dysplasia (D). Note changes of angiogenic squamous dysplasia (ASD) in D.

Clinical characteristics for the biopsies utilized in these studies were obtained from Colorado SPORE in lung cancer survey information collected at or near the time of bronchoscopy. Seven subjects (11 biopsies) were female and 25 subjects (51 biopsies) were male. The age range was 48 – 74 years of age (mean = 68.3). Three biopsies were from subjects who had never smoked while tobacco exposures ranged between 35 and168 pack years for the rest (mean = 55.7 pack years). Thirty-seven biopsies were from subjects that were currently smoking at the time of biopsy and 24 were from previous smokers with an average time of 10.2 years since smoking cessation (range = 1.2 to 32.8 years). A representative subset of twenty biopsies was selected for the analysis of Ang1, Ang2 and Tie2 expression. This set consisted of five normal biopsies, seven low grade dysplasias and eight high grade dysplasias.

Tumor and matched normal tissue derived RNA was collected from resection specimens for which frozen tumor and normal lung from elsewhere in the same specimen had been previously collected and stored in the Colorado SPORE in lung cancer tissue bank. Frozen tissue was removed from storage and a fragment was placed directly into Trizol extraction reagent. RNA was extracted and concentrations measured in the same manner as described above for bronchial biopsies. Matched tumor-normal pairs from thirty-four resections were analyzed for VEGF and angiopoietin/Tie2 expression levels. The tumors were nearly all non-small cell lung cancers and included twelve squamous cell carcinomas, fifteen adenocarcinomas and seven others of various type including one or two examples each of bronchioloalveolar, large cell, pleomorphic and carcinoid tumors. As with the bronchoscopic biopsies, clinical characteristics for the tumor-normal pairs utilized in these studies were obtained from Colorado SPORE in lung cancer survey information collected at or near the time of resection. Fourteen subjects were female and 20 subjects were male. The age range was 34 - 82 years of age (mean = 64.1). Smoking histories were available on only 13 subjects and of these five were never smokers, five were previous smokers and three were current smokers at the time of their resections. The current and previous smokers had associated smoking histories ranging from 6 to 90 pack years with a mean tobacco history of 53.4 pack years. The subjects for whom staging data were available demonstrated a range of pathologic stages including 16 stage I, 9 stage II, 4 stage III and 1 stage IV tumors.

Cultured dysplastic bronchial epithelial cells were derived from the bronchial margin of lung specimens resected for lung cancer or from biopsies taken at bronchoscopy. Biopsy tissue or full sections of bronchus were taken from the fresh resection specimen and transported in bronchial epithelial growth media (BEGM, Cambrex, Walkersville, MD). An immediately adjacent section of bronchus or biopsy tissue adjacent to cultured biopsies was fixed in formalin, embedded in paraffin and subsequently sectioned for hematoxylin and eosin staining. These formalin fixed specimens were used to establish the corresponding histologic classification of the cultured cells. The cultures were established by first incubating the tissue in a dispase solution (Becton-Dickenson, Franklin Lakes, NJ) for one to two hours at 37°C to separate the epithelium from the underlying stromal tissue. Subsequent growth in serum free BEGM allowed for culture of pure bronchial epithelial cells. These cells were grown to confluence and then split 1:4. Once the cells had grown to approximately 50-60% confluence they were trypsinized, counted on a cytometer and frozen in BEGM + 10% DMSO for future use. The cell lines used for *in vitro* endothelial cell assays included four low grade dysplasia and four high grade dysplasia derived cultures.

Endothelial cells used in *in vitro* assays of bronchial dysplasia associated angiogenic activity were derived from human umbilical veins (HUVEC). HUVECs were maintained in RPMI (Mediatech, Herndon, VA) + 10% fetal bovine serum. These cells were a generous gift of Dr. Carlyne Cool, Univeristy of Colorado, Department of Pathology.

## Multiplex, Semi-Quantitative PCR Analysis of Ang1, Ang2 and Tie-2 Expression

A multiplex assay was developed to simultaneously measure levels of Ang1, Ang2 and Tie2 in order to allow multiple measurements in the limited amount of bronchial dysplasia derived RNA available for these studies. This PCR technique was also used to measure Ang1, Ang2 and Tie2 levels in lung cancer and matching normal tissue from resection specimens. For each bronchial biopsy, 1 µg of RNA was reverse transcribed (RT) and 2 µl of the 20 µl RT product was used for the multiplex PCR reaction. In addition, a separate PCR reaction again using 2 µl of RT product was performed to measure actin levels in each specimen so that levels could be normalized for final expression level analysis. The Ang1/Ang2/Tie2 multiplex was developed by performing individual PCR amplification for each of these transcripts in tumor samples over a range of cycle lengths (29 – 37 cycles of PCR). A cycle length that had been shown to be within the logarithmic phase of the amplification curve for all three targets was then chosen for the multiplex reaction which consisted of precycling five minute 94°C step followed by 36 cycles of 94 °C for one minute, 72 °C for one minute and 72 °C for one minute with a final seven minute 74 °C incubation. Validation of the multiplex PCR assay was performed by re-assaying the tumor samples that had been characterized in single PCR reactions in the multiplex assay and close reproduction of the relative levels of the three PCR products in the multiplex PCR reaction as compared to levels found in the single PCR reactions was confirmed. The primers for the three products of the multiplex reaction were chosen such that they could be resolved by separation in subsequent gel electrophoresis. The primers used were as follows: Ang1 ACTGTGCAGATGTATATCAAGC-forward and GTGGAATCTGTCATACTGTGAA-reverse, product 245 bp; Ang2 GGAAGACAAGCACATCATCC-forward and AGTAAGCCTCA TTCCCTTCC-reverse, product 512 bp; Tie2 TCTGTGCTGTTCCTTC TTGC-forward and CTTGAGTAACTTCCAGCGGA-reverse, product 298bp. Actin levels for each specimen were determined in a separate single primer set PCR reaction with GAGGAGCATGATCTTGATCTTC-forward and ATCCACGAAACTACCTTCAACTC-reverse primers that started with a pre-cycling ramp up consisting of 48 °C for 30 minutes, 94 °C for two minutes and 96 °C for three minutes. This was followed by 28 cycles of 94 °C for one minute, 55 °C for one minute and 72 °C for two minutes and a final ten minute 72 °C incubation. PCR products were separated on a 6% denaturing polyacrylamide gel and stained with Vistra Green. Gel images were captured and were analyzed using densitometric measurements produced on a STORM phosphoimaging system. Ang1, Ang2 and Tie2 levels were then normalized via division with similarly determined actin levels for each specimen.

Determination of potential interaction between VEGF and angiopoietin related factors in the production of angiogenic activity was studied by assigning each specimen to an "overexpressor" or "non-overexpressor" group according to the expression of each factor in comparison to the corresponding normal level for a given specimen. Invasive tumors were compared directly to their matched normal tissue from a remote site within the resection specimen. Dysplasias were compared to the average level for each factor determined in the analysis of the normal biopsies as a group. Each specimen was given a score of 1 for over expression or 0 for lack of overexpression for VEGF, Ang1 and Ang2. The sum of these scores was designated as the "angiogenic factor score" for that specimen and used for comparison with the level of angiogenic activity as indicated by the microvessel density (MVD) for that specimen. Because decreased levels of Ang1 have been associated with increased EC proliferation and overexpression of Ang1 has been associated with inhibition of tumor growth in xenograft models, analyses were also done in which a score of one was assigned to specimens with an Ang1 level below the level of corresponding normal tissue. In addition, in order to take into consideration the effect of very high overexpressors or very low non-overexpressors log transformed raw values for the ratio between tumor or dysplasia and normal were used to calculate alternate angiogenic factor scores. Linear regression analysis to test for a relationship between these alternate angiogenic factor scores with MVD were also done. Analyses performed using either angiogenic factor score did not show any differences in respect to statistical significance regarding potential relationships with MVD and data presented for these studies utilize the former angiogenic factor score as described above. The presence of a statistically significant linear trend toward higher MVD in relation to angiogenic factor scores ranging for zero to three was considered to be evidence of a cooperative interaction between the VEGF and angiopoietin pathways. The methods and values used for VEGF levels and MVDs were those previously published for a large subset of the test specimens used in this study [32].

Clinical correlations were tested by two methods. Relationships between factor expression and clinical variables of age and tobacco exposure (pack years) were done by plotting either clinical variable against the expression level of each factor and testing for a statistically significant relationship via linear regression. The clinical variables of gender, smoking status (current, previous or never), tumor stage (tumors only – stage I vs. stage II/III) and nodal metastases (tumors only) were analyzed by comparing differences in t-tests of factor expression levels for specimens assigned to either clinical group.

## *In Vitro* Characterization of Angiogenic Activity

Endothelial cell (EC) proliferation assays were performed using human umbilical vein endothelial cell cultures grown in a 2:1 mixture of endothelial cell growth media (RPMI):bronchial epithelial growth media (BEGM, Cambrex, Walkersville, MD). The EC were plated at $5 \times 10^4$ cells per well in a 24 well plate and serum starved by growth in RPMI plus 2% fetal calf serum for 48 hours prior to addition of conditioned media (CM). CM was collected from bronchial epithelial cells grown in fresh BEGM overnight while at 70-80% confluency. Dysplasia associated induction of EC proliferative activity was assessed by comparing conditioned BEGM (CM) of cells derived from bronchial biopsies taken adjacent to biopsies with documented dysplastic change to EC proliferation test media composed of 2:1 RPMI:unconditioned

BEGM (UCM – negative control). Specificity of VEGF mediatied induction of EC proliferation was established by using a pan-isoform specific neutralizing anti-VEGF antibody (RandD systems, Minneapolis, USA) and an isotype (IgG) matched non-specific immunoglobulin negative control added to CM. A recombinant VEGF165 protein (RandD systems, Minneapolis, USA) was used as positive control in each experiment. VEGF levels were measured in CM via direct ELISA analysis as previously described (32). Each condition was tested in triplicate using three wells on a 24-well plate. After 48 hours of growth in the presence of UCM, UCM + recVEGF, CM, CM + α-VEGF and CM + IgG, cells were immersed in equal volumes of Cyquant fluorescent dye solution (Molecular Probes, Eugene, OR, USA) for two to five minutes. This solution lyses endothelial cells and binds to DNA in a stoichiometric fashion giving a fluorescent signal that can be measured on a STORM phosphoimager. Relative EDC proliferation was compared between test groups by performing T-tests to determine statistically significant differences between groups.

Endothelial cell migration assays were performed in a manner similar to that used for endothelial cell proliferation. However, these assays utilized 12 well multiwell plates with .45 μm pore size membrane equipped inserts onto which $5x10^5$ EC were plated in ECGM with 2% FBS. After overnight culture of the endothelial cells to allow for attachment, the cultures were switched to serum free ECGM and UCM and CM with the same supplements as described for the proliferation assay above were placed in the wells underlying the endothelial cell seeded inserts. Migration of endothelial cells into the wells underlying the inserts was allowed to proceed for 24 hours. The inserts were then removed, the cells were stained with Trypan blue and four representative fields within each well were tallied using an inverted microscope.

Assessment of the capacity of dysplasia derived CM to induce endothelial cell tubule formation was also performed. This tubulogenesis assay was performed using 24 well culture plates in which 100 μl of Matrigel (Becton Dickinson Labware, Bedford, MA) per well were placed and allowed to set for 30 minutes at $37^o$ C. $3 \times 10^4$ cells were then seeded onto these matrigel substructures and the cells were then serum starved in .5% serum supplemented RPMI overnight. The media was changed the next day and 500 μl of 1:2 CM:RPMI+.5% serum was added to the wells. The test groups, as described above, were tested in triplicate and results were evaluated after a 24 hour incubation in test media in two representative fields per well as captured in digital images. Image analysis provided measurements of number and length of tubules formed, and was performed using ImagePro software to tag tubule structures for tallying tubule sprouting and calculate tubule lengths employing a specifically calibrated linear tracing tool.

ELISA analysis of VEGF levels was performed on CM and on extracted proteins from tumor tissue specimens. Protein was extracted by homogenizing frozen tissue in 1 ml of RIPA buffer (50mM Tris, 150 mM NaCl, 2mM EDTA, 50 mM NaF, 1% Triton X-100, 1% sodium deoxycholate, .1% SDS, 1mM DTT and 5mM sodium orthovanadate) supplemented with a protease inhibitor cocktail (Sigma, St. Louis, MO) and then centrifuging at 15,000g at 4°C for 20 minutes. Total protein was measured for each specimen utilizing a Bio-Rad DC protein assay system. Thawed proteins were washed in 100% ethanol and resuspended for analysis in a phosphate buffered saline solution containing .5% sodium dodecyl sulfate.

### Statistical Analysis

The primary analyses focused on characterization of angiopoietin expression in dysplastic and tumor tissue and on *in vitro* studies of VEGF mediated angiogenic activity. For these studies a t-test of the difference between expression levels in lesional versus normal tissues were performed. Secondary analyses addressed the association of combined angiogenic factor effects on angiogenic activity as measured by MVD and the relationship between factor expression and a number of clinical characteristics associated with each subject. Linear regression models and chi-square analyses were used to estimate and test the significance of correlations between these parameters. Results are reported as 2-sided p-values.

## RESULTS

### Subject Population

Bronchial dysplasias and paired tumor-normal specimens were all sorted according primary clinical characteristics of age, gender and smoking history to determine if differences in expression levels of VEGF, Ang1, Ang2 or Tie2 were confounded by a relationship between expression of these factors and the noted characteristics. VEGF expression levels in dysplasias were not associated with significant differences related to age, gender or smoking history except for the previously noted significant trend toward higher expression of VEGF in histologically normal biopsies from smokers with greater than 50 pack year smoking histories as compared to normal biopsies from smokers with lesser exposure [32, data not shown]. This trend was not seen in dypslastic lesions from subjects assigned to the same smoking history groups. Similarly, the subset of dysplasias that were analyzed for angiopoietin expression showed no association between age, gender or smoking histories and levels of expression of Ang1, Ang2 and Tie2. However, given the limited number of specimens used in this analysis (20 biopsies) some relationships may not have been detected especially in respect to gender where only two female subjects were included.

Paired tumor-normal specimens showed no statistically significant differences in expression of VEGF related to subject age, gender or smoking history. In respect to expression of Ang1, Ang2 and Tie2, linear regression analysis showed no statistically significant differences related to subject age or smoking history. Of note however, was the detection of a statistically a significant increase in expression of Ang1 and Tie 2 in normal tissue from female subjects as compared to normal tissue from male subjects (data not shown). This difference was not seen in tumor tissues segregated according to gender.

## Expression of Angiopoietin 1 and 2 and Their Receptor, Tie2 in Bronchial Dysplasia and Invasive Non-Small Cell Lung Carcinomas

Actin normalized expression levels of Ang1, Ang2 and Tie2 were measured for five histologically normal bronchial biopsies and fifteen bronchial dysplasias (7 low-grade and 8 high-grade). In comparison to normal, bronchial dysplasias did not show statistically significant alterations of Ang1, Ang2 or Tie2 expression (figure 2A). Although a trend toward increased expression of Ang2 was noted, this did not reach statistical significance ($p = 0.130$). Comparisons of expression levels in low-grade and high-grade dysplasias taken separately showed no differences between these two groups or between either group and normal bronchial mucosa (data not shown).

Lung carcinomas showed significantly decreased levels of Ang1 and Tie2 expression as compared to matched normal tissue (figure 2B). Ang2 levels were not different between tumor tissues and matched normal lung. Tumors were also analyzed to determine whether expression levels of angiopoietin

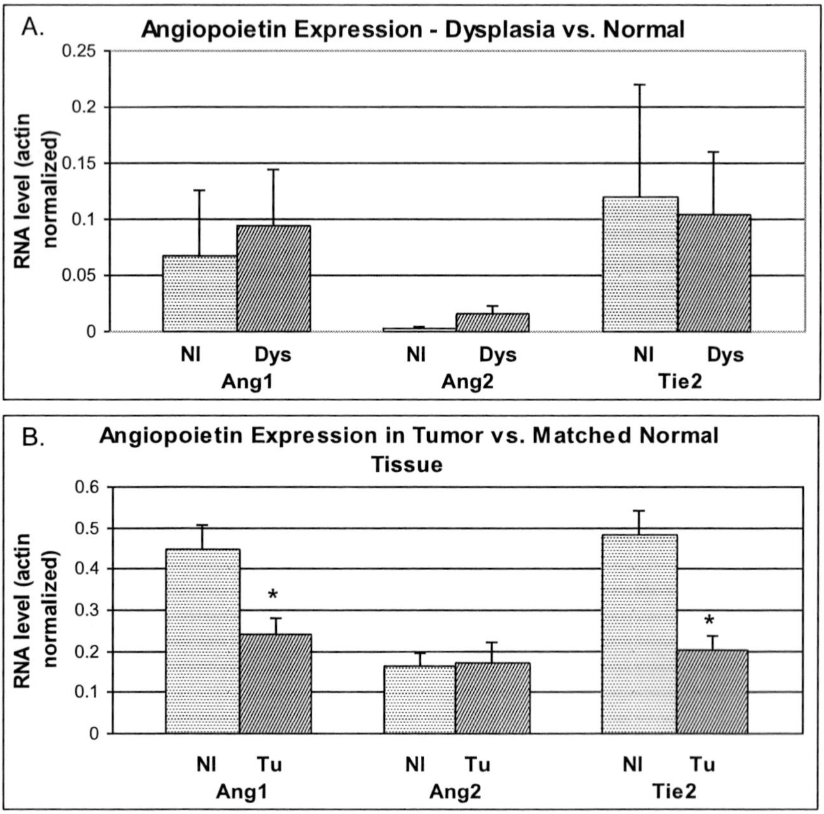


Figure 2. Graphs showing (A) absence of statistically significant alteration of Ang1, Ang2 and Tie2 expression levels in bronchial dysplasia as compared to normal bronchial epithelium, and (B) presence of statistically significant (*) decreases in Ang1 ($p = 0.006$) and Tie2 ($p < 0.001$) but not Ang2 in tumor tissue as compared to normal . Bars show standard error of mean.

family members were associated with prognostic characteristics. Tumors with documented lymph node metastases did not show any statistically significant differences of Ang1, Ang2 or Tie2 expression levels when compared to those without known lymph node metastases.

In addition linear regression analyses did not show statistically significant correlations between Ang1, Ang2 or Tie2 expression levels and tumor stage or tumor size (data not shown). Given the significant number of squamous cell carcinomas and adenocarcinomas in our study set, we also analyzed these separately and found that while adenocarcinomas paralleled the findings for the tumor-normal set as a whole, squamous cell carcinomas did not maintain a statistically significant difference in Ang1 levels as compared to their matched normal tissue though a trend toward lower expression was present (data not shown). Decreased Tie2 expression was found in squamous cell carcinomas also. There were no statistically significant differences in expression of these factors when adenocarcinomas were compared to squamous cell carcinomas.

## Combined Analysis of VEGF and Angiopoietin Expression in Relation to Angiogenic Activity in Bronchial Dysplasia and Invasive Lung Carcinoma

Data regarding angiopoietin expression was combined with previously published data on VEGF expression and microvessel densities for the specimens analyzed in this chapter to determine if a cooperative effect could be demonstrated between these two pathways in respect to induction of angiogenic activity. As described in the materials and methods section, each specimen was given a score of 1 for over expression or 0 for lack of overexpression for VEGF, Ang1 and Ang2 and the sum of these scores, the "angiogenic factor score," was used for comparison with the level of angiogenic activity as indicated by the microvessel density for that specimen. Dysplasias were given scores for VEGF, Ang1 and Ang2 based on the expression level in the specimen as compared to the average level of expression for that factor in the entire group of histologically normal biopsies. Linear regression analysis of angiogenic factor score versus MVD did not demonstrate a statistically significant relationship in bronchial dypslasia (table 2A). In addition, when dysplasias were analyzed as individual groups of low-grade or high-grade lesions, no significant relationship existed (data not shown). Tumors were scored for overexpression of VEGF, Ang1 and Ang2 in direct comparison with the levels of expression of the factor in their matched normal tissue. Angiogenic factor scores were calculated in a manner identical to that described for dysplasia above. The data were analyzed via linear regression plotting angiogenic factor scores against MVDs and also showed no significant relationship between these parameters in invasive tumors (table 2B). However, a particularly interesting observation was seen in the bronchial biopsy group when an analysis of MVD versus VEGF overexpression score alone was performed. Statistically significant increases in MVD were seen in biopsies with VEGF overexpression when compared to those without (figure 3, $p = 0.031$). MVDs were not different in the normal/RCH group or the low grade dysplasia group when analyzed individually, but high grade dysplasias

**Table 2. Correlation between angiogenic factor expression and microvessel density**

| | AFS =0[1] | AFS=1 | AFS=2 | AFS=3 | |
|---|---|---|---|---|---|
| | Avg. MVD[2] Vessels/mm$^2$ | Avg. MVD Vessels/mm$^2$ | Avg. MVD Vessels/mm$^2$ | Avg. MVD Vessels/mm$^2$ | P-value[3] |
| A) Dysplasia: | | | | | |
| | 105.6 (2)[4] | 88.7 (3) | 103.9 (5) | 51.1 (1) | 0.329 |
| | | | | | |
| B) Tumor: | | | | | |
| | 778.0 (2) | 470.5 (14) | 232.8 (3) | 682.3 (4) | 0.937 |
| | | | | | |

[1]AFS = angiogenic factor score. AFS calculated as the sum of overexpression scores for VEGF, Ang1 and Ang2 where overexpression = 1 and non-overexpression = 0. [2]MVD is microvessel density. [3]P-value test for linear trends across AFS groups. [4]N for each AFS group.

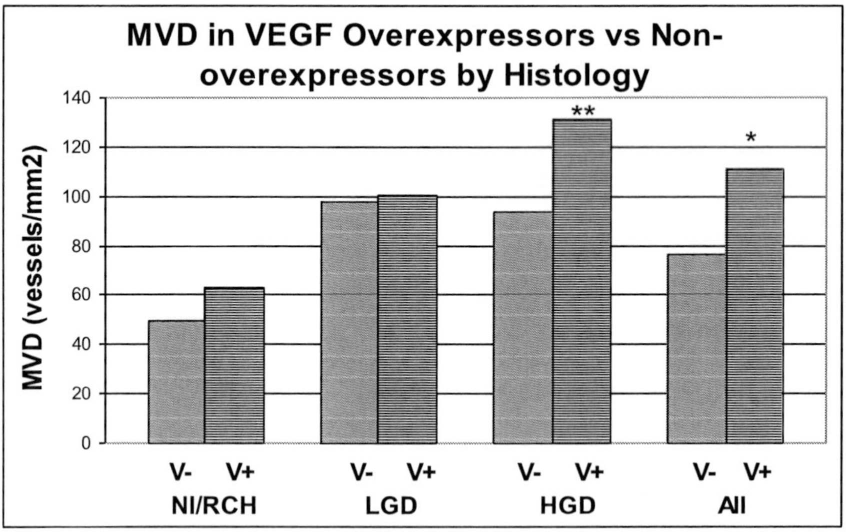


Figure 3. Graph demonstrating association between overexpression of VEGF (V+) and increased microvessel density (MVD) as compared to non-overexpressors (V-) (*p < 0.05). Normal/reserve cell hyperplasia (Nl/RCH) and low grade dysplasia (LGD) groups show no association between VEGF overexpression and increased MVD, but high grade dysplasias (HGD) show a strong trend toward increased MVD with VEGF overexpressin (**p = 0.062).

**Table 3. Correlation between VEGF expression and clinical tumor characteristics**

| | VEGF RNA | | | VEGF Protein | | |
|---|---|---|---|---|---|---|
| | OE[1] | No OE | p-value[2] | OE | No OE | p-value |
| | | | | | | |
| >2 LN[3] Mets: | 5/5 | 0/5 | 0.041 | 4/5 | 1/5 | 0.433 |
| 0-1 LN Mets: | 10/20 | 10/20 | | 11/18 | 7/18 | |
| | | | | | | |
| Stage 2/3: | 9/10 | 1/10 | 0.045 | 5/10 | 5/10 | 0.225 |
| Stage 1: | 6/12 | 6/12 | | 3/12 | 9/12 | |
| | | | | | | |
| Tumor >3cm: | 10/14 | 4/14 | 0.188 | 6/12 | 6/12 | 0.342 |
| Tumor <3cm: | 5/11 | 6/11 | | 7/10 | 3/10 | |
| | | | | | | |
| VI[4] Present: | 3/5 | 2/5 | 0.970 | 1/4 | 3/4 | 0.090 |
| VI Absent: | 13/22 | 9/22 | | `4/10 | 6/10 | |

[1] OE = Overexpression. Overexpression is determined by comparison to VEGF levels in corresponding normal tissue for each specimen. [2]P-value determined by chi-square analysis. [3]LN = Lymph node. [4]VI = Vascular invasion.

showed a strong trend toward significant elevation of MVD in VEGF overexpressors as compared to non-overexpressors (figure 3, p =0.062). VEGF overexpression in tumors was not associated with a significant increase in MVD when considered alone. Similar analyses of each Ang1, Ang2 and Tie2 alone did not show a relationship between overexpression and MVD in dysplasias or tumors.

An analysis was also performed to determine if there was a relationship between expression of VEGF and angiopoietin family members and clinical characteristics of disease for the invasive tumors. When tumors were classified as VEGF RNA overexpressors or non-overexpressors, chi-square analyses revealed a statistically significant association of VEGF overexpression with the presence of multiple lymph node metastases and with stage II or higher tumors versus stage I disease (table 3). These relationships were not found when assessing VEGF protein levels and neither VEGF RNA or protein overexpression were associated with increased incidence of vascular invasion or tumor size (data not shown). Similarly, no statistically significant relationship between expression levels of Ang1, Ang2 or Tie2 and tumor stage, lymph node metastasis or tumor size were found (data not shown).

## *In Vitro* Characterization of Dysplasia and Tumor Derived Angiogenic Activity: Mechanistic Role of VEGF

Endothelial cell proliferation assays employing conditioned media collected from cultures of six bronchial dysplasias and five invasive NSCLCs were used to test their ability to stimulate endothelial cell proliferation *in vitro*. In comparison to unconditioned media, statistically significant increases in EC proliferation were noted in five of six assays performed with conditioned media from bronchial dysplasia and in five of five assays performed with conditioned media from invasive NSCLCs (representative experiments shown in figure 4A and B). Addition of a pan-isoform specific neutralizing antibody against VEGF was used to establish specificity between conditioned media induced proliferative responses and dysplasia or carcinoma associated VEGF production. Complete abrogation of this proliferative response, as indicated by reduction of EC proliferation to levels that were not significantly different than that seen in unconditioned media (UCM), was demonstrated in four of five dysplasias but only one of five NSCLCs. Addition of a non-specific, isotype matched antibody did not alter the proliferative response induced by conditioned media in any of the assays. VEGF levels in the conditioned media were measured by ELISA analysis of aliquots taken from the conditioned media used in the EC proliferation assays for all cell lines tested. Average levels of VEGF in bronchial dysplasia derived conditioned media was 67.1 pg/ml and NSCLC conditioned media demonstrated average levels of 210.6 pg/ml. Finally, regression analysis was performed in plots of VEGF levels versus degree of EC proliferation, as indicated by the CM:UCM ratios to further verify the mechanistic role of dysplasia or carcinoma derived VEGF in the induction of this response. Similarly, this analysis revealed a close correlation between dysplasia VEGF levels and degree of EC proliferation ($R^2 = 0.6386$, $p = 0.056$) and poor correlation between NSCLC VEGF levels and degree of EC proliferation ($R^2 = 0.1282$, $p = 0.55$) (figure 4C).

Endothelial cell migration was analyzed by testing the capacity of conditioned media from seven dysplasia derived cell lines to stimulate translocation of EC from well inserts with .45 μm pore membranes into underlying wells of 12 well culture plates in which the conditioned media had been placed. Six of seven dysplasias showed statistically significant induction of EC migration as compared to migration in the presence of UCM (figure 5).

Addition of neutralizing anti-VEGF antibody to the conditioned media of the six cell lines that induced migration reduced this effect to basal migration levels in four of them (i.e. not statistically different than UCM).

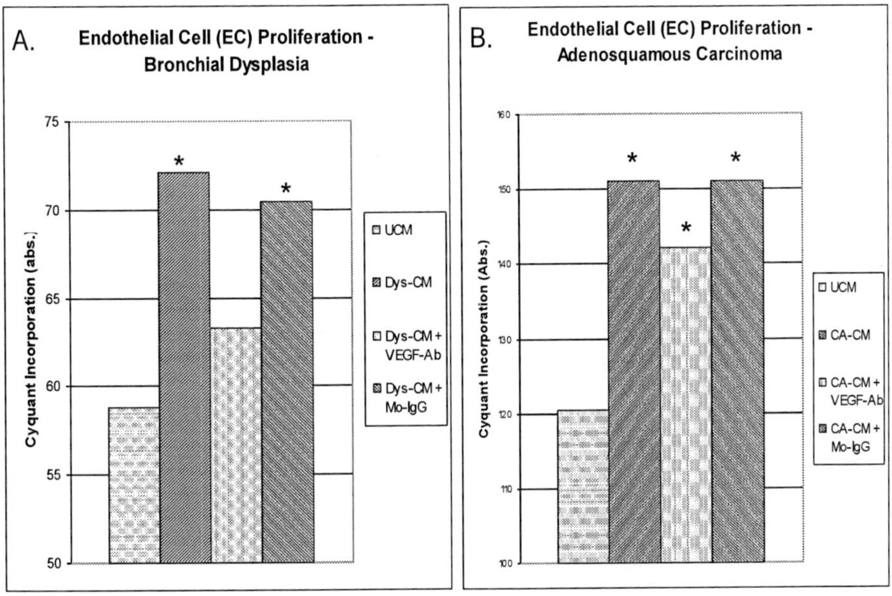


C.

| | CM>UCM* | UCM= CM+αVEGF* | Avg CM VEGF protein (pg/ml) | $R^2$ VEGF vs. CM:UCM ratio* |
|---|---|---|---|---|
| Dysplasia | 5/6 | 4/5 | 67.1 | 0.6386 |
| Tumor | 5/5 | 1/5 | 210.6 | 0.1282 |

Figure 4. *In vitro* endothelial cell proliferation assays. A) Representative analysis of bronchial dysplasia derived conditioned media (Dys-CM) mediated induction of EC proliferation (*$p < 0.05$) as compared to unconditioned media (UCM). Non-specific antibody (Dys-CM + Mo-IgG) does not inhibit the effect whereas VEGF specific antibody (Dys-CM + VEGF-Ab) abrogates significant induction. B) Representative analysis showing similar effect of tumor derived conditioned media on EC proliferation with exception of incomplete abrogation of effect by addition of VEGF specific antibody. C) Table summarizing results from EC proliferation assays of multiple dysplasia and tumor derived conditioned media (*$p < 0.05$ to meet criteria for columns one and two). Conditioned media VEGF protein levels as measured in ELISA analyses are shown in the third column and results of linear regression analyses comparing VEGF levels to the ratio of conditioned media and unconditioned media for the group of dysplasia and tumor derived specimens are shown in the fourth column (*, $p = 0.056$ for dysplasia and $p = 0.554$ for tumor).

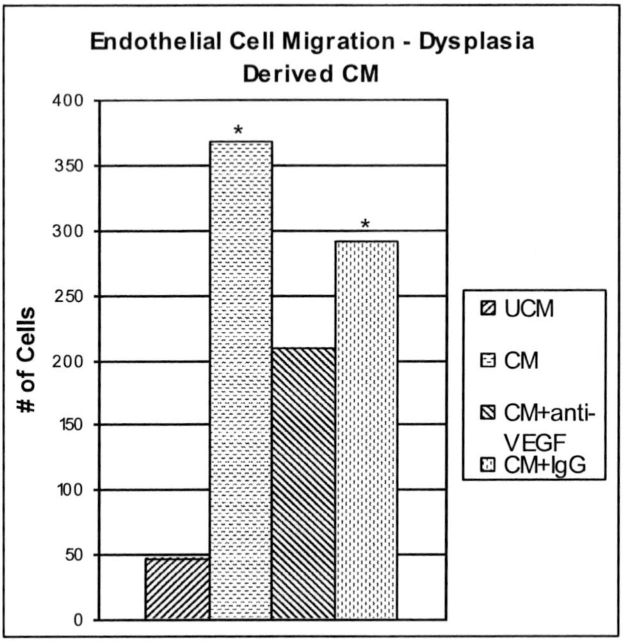


Figure 5. In vitro assay of endothelial cell migration in presence of conditioned media (CM) from cultured dypslastic bronchial epithelium. Statistically significant increase in endothelial cell migration in seen in CM and CM plus neutralizing VEGF antibody (CM+anti-VEGF) but not CM plus control antibody (CM+IgG) (*p<0.05).

*In vitro* endothelial cell tubulogenesis assays were used to measure the ability of conditioned media to induce tubule elongation (tubule length) and vessel branching (tubule sprouts) in an assay utilizing EC seeded on a matrigel matrix. Representative digital images from wells grown in the presence of unconditioned media, dysplasia conditioned media and dysplasia conditioned media with added neutralizing antibody to VEGF are shown in figure 6. Conditioned media from five of six dysplasia derived and five of five NSCLC derived cell lines demonstrated statistically significant induction of tubule elongation as compared to unconditioned media (figure 7A and C). All conditioned media that induced tubule elongation could be fully inhibited by addition of neutralizing anti-VEGF antibody. Tubule sprouting was induced relative to unconditioned media by only one of three NSCLC cell lines and none of the six dysplasia cell lines (figure 7B and C). The single tumor cell line that was able to induce an increase in tubule sprout formation was fully inhibited by the addition of neutralizing anti-VEGF antibody.

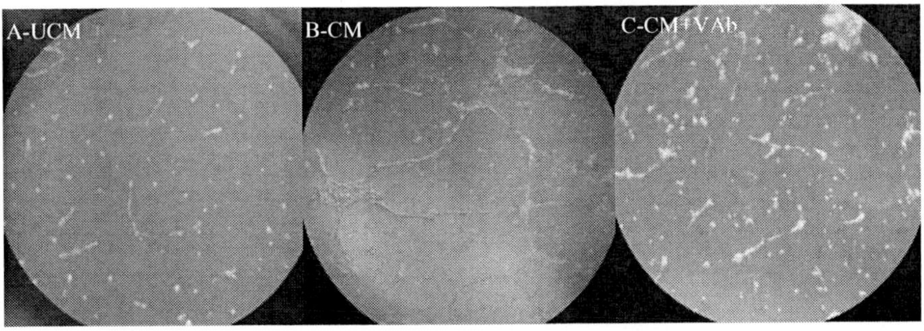


Figure 6. Representative fields from an endothelial cell tubulogenesis assay grown in unconditioned media (A-UCM), dysplasia conditioned media (B-CM) and conditioned media supplemented with neutralizing anti-VEGF antibody (C-CM+VAb). Although similar number of tubules are seen in A and B, the length of the tubules is significantly increased and this effect is blocked by addition of anti-VEGF.

**Table 4. Summary of findings for in vitro assays of endothelial cell proliferation, migration and tubulogenesis using conditioned media from cultures of dysplastic bronchial epithelial cells**

| | CM>UCM* | UCM= CM+αVEGF** | Avg CM VEGF protein (pg/ml) | $R^2$ VEGF vs. CM:UCM ratio* |
|---|---|---|---|---|
| EDC proliferation | 5/6 | 4/5 | 67.1 | 0.6386 |
| EDC migration | 6/7 | 4/6 | ND | ND |
| Tubule length | 5/6 | 5/5 | ND | ND |
| Tubule formation | 0/6 | NA | ND | ND |

Specificity of VEGF mediated effect is indicated by UCM =CM+anti-VEGF column where **p>0.05. *p<0.05 for columns one and four.

Table 4 summarizes the *in vitro* characterization of dysplasia VEGF associated angiogenic activity. The results show that there is near ubiquitous induction of the EC activities that characterize the proliferative phase of angiogenesis including EC proliferation, EC migration and tubule elongation. In addition nearly all of the cell lines that induce these activities can be completely inhibited by the addition of a VEGF neutralizing antibody establishing the specificity of VEGF mediated induction and indicating that VEGF plays a central mechanistic role in stimulating proliferative angiogenic activity in bronchial dysplasia. Notably, tubule sprout formation, the single measure of maturational/differentiative angiogenic activity assayed in these studies, is not induced by any of the dysplasia derived cells lines.

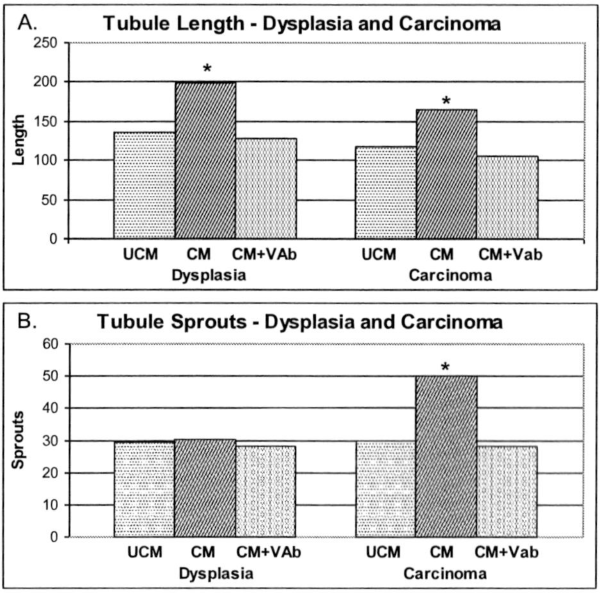


C.

| | | CM>UCM* | UCM= CM+αVEGF* |
|---|---|---|---|
| Dysplasia | Tubule Length | 5/6 | 5/5 |
| | Tubule Sprouts | 0/6 | NA |
| Tumor | Tubule Length | 3/3 | 3/3 |
| | Tubule Sprouts | 1/3 | 1/1 |

Figure 7. *In vitro* endothelial cell tubulogenesis assays. A) Representative analysis showing induction of tubule length by dysplasia and tumor derived conditioned media (CM) as compared to unconditioned media (UCM). VEGF specific antibody (CM + VAb) abrogates significant induction for both dypslasia and tumor. B) Representative analysis showing similar effect of tumor but not dysplasia derived conditioned media on tubule sprout formation. C) Table summarizing results from tubulogenesis assays of multiple dysplasia and tumor derived CM (*$p < 0.05$).

## DISCUSSION

Angiogenesis is a hallmark of lung cancer and malignancies in general, and our previous work has demonstrated that angiogenic activity and increased VEGF expression are also present in bronchial dysplasia [32]. Invasive lung cancer has been convincingly shown to be associated with alterations in the expression of several angiogenic mediators and this led to the supposition that other angiogenic factors might contribute to aniogenic activity in bronchial dysplasia as well. Therefore, an analysis of the expression of angiopoietins Ang1 and Ang2 and their receptor Tie2 in bronchial dysplasia was performed. The results failed to show significant alterations in the expression of any of these factors when comparing bronchial dysplasias to histologically normal bronchial epithelium. Furthermore, a variety of techniques were applied to determine if a cooperative effect between VEGF and angiopoietin might act as a primary determinant of angiogenic activity in bronchial dysplasia. No relationship was found between combined VEGF-angiopoietin expression profiles and MVDs in these lesions.

Invasive lung carcinomas, on the other hand, did demonstrate decreased Ang1 and Tie2 expression in comparison to normal lung. Although previous studies of lung cancer have produced some conflicting results, these findings are in agreement with several other studies of Ang1 and Tie2 in lung cancer [21,22]. In addition to these previously noted alterations in Ang1 and Tie2 expresion in lung cancer, a number of observations have found Ang2 to be elevated in lung cancers. Our results did not find any difference in Ang2 expression levels in tumors as compared to normal lung. This discrepancy may simply be related to a lack of adequate numbers of specimens to demonstrate such a difference in our study, but our data did not show any trend toward increased Ang2 in tumors. Indeed, it has been suggested that the primary role of Ang2 may be to act as an antagonist of Ang1 [15], and therefore its overexpression may not be of significant importance when Ang1 levels and expression of its receptor Tie2 are significantly decreased as we found. Some functional implications that are likely of significant importance in the progression of lung carcinomas can be attributed to decreased Ang1 and Tie2 expression. As discussed earlier, angiopoietin activity induces the recruitment of pericytes and promotes mural vessel wall maturation. A number of studies have now correlated the absence of pericytic influx and vascular maturation with an increased risk for the development of metastases [35,36]. Therefore, the presence of decreased Ang1 and Tie2 expression in lung carcinomas would favor tumor progression. In respect to dysplastic lesions of the bronchial airways, the capacity to metastasize is not a characteristic that would provide these lesions with a significant advantage given the early stage of development they occupy in the progression of lung cancer.

While our results seem to support the concept that a complex network of angiogenic factors orchestrate angiogenic activity in invasive lung cancers, the absence of altered angiopoietin expression in dysplasias provided little information regarding the overall control of angiogenesis in these lesions. However, the demonstration of an association between VEGF overexpression and increased MVD in bronchial tissue has opened the possibility that VEGF may be adequate to stimulate the amount and type of angiogenic activity necessary for the development of these lesions. Furthermore, the finding of a trend toward this association in high grade dysplasias in conjunction with the absence of such an association in normal/reactive (reserve cell hyperplasia) epithelium and low grade dysplasia suggests that VEGF overexpression may play an important role in the progression of bronchial dysplasia. Indeed, several observations from our initial characterization of VEGF expression in bronchial dysplasia lend support to the concept of VEGF as the central mediator of angiogenesis in this disease. While VEGF was elevated in all dysplasias as compared to normal, it was most prominently expressed in the subset of dysplastic lesions that show histologic evidence of angiogenesis, the angiogenic squamous dysplasias (ASD). This histologic feature is relatively frequent in dysplastic disease of the airways and has been shown to persist in subjects undergoing repeat bronchoscopy [33]. Another feature of ASDs described in our previous study is the presence of increased expression of VEGF receptors including VEGF-R2 (KDR). We also demonstrated that in comparison to normal lung tissue, bronchial dysplasias and early stage lung carcinomas showed a shift toward expression of the VEGF121 isoform over the VEGF 165 isoform of VEGF ligand. This isoform profile was not seen in advanced lung cancer. The VEGF121 isoform has relatively complete restriction of specificity for the VEGF-R2 receptor and its interaction with VEGF-R2 is considered to be one of the primary pathways for induction of proliferative endothelial cell responses. Taken together, this combination of VEGF isoform and receptor expression patterns would suggest that VEGF signaling in bronchial dysplasias is oriented toward the proliferative phase of angiogenic activity.

The *in vitro* endothelial cell assays were performed to document a mechanistic link between increased VEGF expression and angiogenic effects in bronchial dysplasia. In addition, measurements of multiple activities allowed us to more thoroughly evaluate the overall character of dysplasia associated angiogenesis in respect to proliferative and maturational actions. Endothelial cell activities associated with the proliferative phase of angiogenesis including proliferation, migration and tubule elongation were elevated in nearly all of the dysplasia derived cell lines analyzed. Conversely, none of the dysplasia derived cell lines showed significant increases in the formation of new tubule sprouts, an activity classically associated with the maturational phase of angiogenesis [3,4]. Furthermore, for the cell lines that did show induction of proliferative endothelial cell activities, complete abrogation of this activity by inclusion of a pan-isoform anti-VEGF neutralizing antibody was nearly ubiquitous with 5/6, 4/6 and 5/5 cell lines demonstrating reduction to basal levels of proliferation, migration and tubule elongation, respectively. Finally, when we compared levels of VEGF present in the conditioned media used in these assays with the ratio of proliferation in dysplasia conditioned media as compared to unconditioned media, we found a strong correlation between VEGF level and degree of increase in endothelial cell proliferation. These latter findings establish a strong relationship between VEGF expression and the induction of these proliferative angiogenic activities. Future studies of interest would include *in vitro* assays in which VEGF isoform and receptor specific inhibitors would be added to dysplasia derived conditioned media allowing for the identification of the primary mediators of VEGF induced angiogenic activity in these lesions. Results from analyses such as these would provide important information in regard to identifying inhibitors of the VEGF pathway with the greatest potential for clinical utility in lung cancer chemoprevention. Additionally, such studies may help identify biomarkers that would not only be specific for bronchial dysplasia but might also give prognostic information regarding potential for progression in dysplastic lesions.

We were also able to compare the angiogenic characteristics described for dysplasias to those found in assays of conditioned media from invasive lung cancer derived cell lines. All tumor derived conditioned media analyzed showed induction of endothelial proliferation and tubule elongation. However, abrogation of proliferation by addition of neutralizing VEGF antibody was accomplished in only one of the five tumor cell lines tested. This finding suggests that additional angiogenic factors are frequently present in invasive tumors in contrast to the results found with dysplasias. Only three tumor cell lines were tested for tubule sprout formation and two of those were negative. While difficult to interpret as a single finding, the identification of a tumor cell line that did induce tubule sprout formation is intriguing. Of note also in respect to this specimen was the fact that anti-VEGF antibody fully blocked this increase in tubule sprout formation. This may indicate that the VEGF isoforms and receptors active in at least some invasive lung cancer differ significantly from those in bronchial dysplasias such that they can promote maturational angiogenic activity. Given the large size that invasive carcinomas can attain, focal maturational phase type angiogenic activity might be advantageous in that it could provide a mature vascular network with consistent nutrient delivery.

Overall our results suggest that angiogenic activity in bronchial dysplasia is distinct from that seen in invasive carcinoma and normal reactive processes. It appears that VEGF may be more prominent in dysplasia associated angiogenesis than it is in invasive carcinomas and in this respect it is possible that control of angiogenic activity in bronchial dysplasia occurs via a simpler mechanism. The results also indicate that a proliferative type of angiogenic response is emphasized in bronchial dysplasia. While this also appears to be the case in invasive carcinomas, the maintenance of a proliferative angiogenic state in tumors may require involvement of more angiogenic pathways as evidenced by the significant decreases in Ang1 and Tie2 expression described in this chapter. The frequent overexpression of VEGF and the general presence of increased microvessel densities in bronchial dysplasia have established that angiogenesis is active in these lesions and suggests that it plays an important role in their development. Supporting this latter point are our data showing that as histologic atypia increases there is an increasing correlation between VEGF overexpression and angiogenic activity as indicated in MVD measurements. A number of previous publications have provided evidence that the malignant potential associated with dysplastic bronchial lesions increases with increasing degrees of atypia. Dysplasias and carcinoma in-situ (CIS) demonstrate features of true premalignant lesions with studies documenting the development of carcinoma in 10 – 40% of patients with moderate and severe dysplasia by sputum cytology [37,38]. The majority of a small group of patients with biopsy proven CIS progressed to invasive carcinoma in clinical follow-up [38,39]. Thus, a correlation between development of angiogenic activity and degree of dysplastic change such as that demonstrated here could suggest that the development of angiogenic activity is important in the progression of these lesions.

The importance of angiogenesis to the development and progression of dysplastic squamous lesions is further supported by a few recent reports showing similar findings in other epithelial tissues. In dysplasia of the uterine cervix (cervical intraepithelial neoplasia/CIN), increased levels of VEGF expression have been found and a relationship between the degree of histologic atypia and level of VEGF has been demonstrated [40]. Similarly, increased expression of VEGF and an association between the frequency of VEGF expression and degree of atypia has been seen in oral squamous dysplasia [41,42]. In addition, levels of VEGF expression in uterine cervix have been shown to correlate with microvessel density much the same as we have demonstrated herein [43]. Of note in regard to angiogenesis in cervical dysplasia is a study that demonstrated a relationship between PDECGF expression and degree of atypia, but did not find such a relationship with VEGF expression [44]. These results are a reminder that a number of angiogenic factors can affect angiogenesis and that the possibility that other factors may contribute angiogenesis in dysplasias must be considered. Approximately 10-20% of the cell lines we tested in *in vitro* endothelial cell assays showed induction of endothelial cell proliferation, migration or tubule elongation that was only partially inhibited by addition of neutralizing VEGF antibody. Additional studies of non-VEGF angiogenic factors that could synergize or substitute for VEGF in producing angiogenic activity in bronchial and other dysplasias is warranted.

If angiogenesis is contributing to the development and progression of dysplastic lesions of the bronchial tree and other epithelia as we have suggested, what is the mechanism by which it makes this contribution? Certainly the answer to this question is based in speculation, but a number of recent observations may hold some clues. Given the commonly held belief that tumors can grow to sizes of approximately .4 mm without any demonstrable angiogenic activity, the importance of angiogenic activity in premalignant lesions has been questioned. Provision of adequate nutrients to support a high level of epithelial proliferation may be critically important to establishing dysplastic lesions and promoting progression of these lesions. The multi-step theory of carcinogenesis has become widely established as the primary driving force behind the development of malignant disease in numerous tissues. Maintaining a high level of epithelial proliferation would allow for the more frequent accumulation of genetic alterations associated with the progression of malignant processes and would help establish clones of highly transformed cells in tissues undergoing the transition from pre-malignant to invasive disease. The proliferative phase of angiogenesis is ideal in this capacity because it provides a significantly greater area of vascular supply for increasingly cellular overlying dysplastic epithelia and enhances nutrient delivery via high permeability of the newly established vasculature. Another possible contribution of angiogenesis to the development of dysplasias relates to the presence of high vascular permeability in neovascular blood vessels.

Previous work has established that VEGF can lead to increased vesicle and leaky junction mediated permeability in endothelial cells [45,46. This permeability may contribute to the progression of cells undergoing malignant transformation by providing access to endogenous and exogenous substances that can promote this transformation. A recent study of the breast cancer cell line, MCF7 has demonstrated that vector mediated expression of the transcription factor twist leads to increased elaboration of VEGF from this cell line. When tumor xenografts grown in mice with this VEGF producing cell line are compared to tumors grown with unaltered MCF7 cells, they show significantly increased vascular permeability that correlates with high grade behavior and associated increased chromosomal instability [47].

In summary, our results demonstrate bronchial dysplasia associated angiogenic activity that appears to be primarily proliferative in nature and predominantly mediated by VEGF. These findings suggest that angiogenic activity may be important to the development and progression of bronchial dysplasia and may hold prognostic significance in these lesions. Additional studies of dysplasia associated angiogenesis hold the promise of identifying targets for effective lung cancer chemoprevention and could provide biomarkers of this disease that may be useful in diagnostic and predictive clinical assays.

## REFERENCES

[1] Hanahan D and Folkman J. Patterns and emerging mechanisms of the angiogenic switch during tumorigensis. *Cell.* 1996 86,353-64.

[2] Soker S, Takashima S, Miao HQ, Neufeld G, Klagsbrun M. Neuropilin-1 is expressed by endothelial and tumor cells as an isoform-specific receptor for vascular endothelial growth factor. *Cell.* 1998 92,735-45.

[3] Bussolati B, Dunk C, Grohman M, Kontos CD, Mason J, Ahmed A. Vascular endothelial growth factor receptor-1 modulates vascular endothelial growth factor-mediated angiogenesis via nitric oxide. *Am. J. Pathol.* 2001 159,993-1008,.

[4] Rahimi N, Dayanir V and Lashkar K. Receptor chimeras indicate that the vascular endothelial growth facto receptor-1 (VEGFR-1) modulates mitogenic activity of VEGFR-2 in endothelial cells. *J. Biol. Chem.* 2000 275,16986-16992.

[5] Meyer RD, Rahimi N. Comparative structure-function analysis of VEGFR-1 and VEGFR-2. *Ann. NY Acac. Sci.* 2003 995,200-7.

[6] Cherng JM, Lin CM, Lin CL, Huang SM, Chang HL, Lee CC, Chiang LC, Chang PY. Effects of VEGF121 and/or VEGF165 gene transfection on collateral circulation development. *J. Formos. Med. Assoc.* 2000 99,603-11.

[7] Meyer RD, Latz C, Rahimi N. Recruitment and activation of phospholipase Cγ1by vascular endothelial growth factor receptor-2 are required for tubulogenesis and differentiation of endothelial cells. *J. Biol. Chem.* 2003 278,16347-55.

[8] Ono M, Okamura K, Nakayama Y, Tomita M, Sato Y, Komatsu Y, Kuwano M. Induction of human microvascular endothelial tubular morphogenesis by human keratinocytes: involvement of TGF-□. *Biochem. Biophys. Res. Commun.* 1992 15,601-609.

[9] Tian S, Hayes AJ, Metheny-Barlow LJ and Li LY. Stabilization of breast cancer xenograft tumour neovasculature by angiopoietin-1. *Br. J. Cancer* 2002 86(4), 645-51.

[10] Iurlaro M, Scatena M, Zhu WH, Fogel E, Wieting SL and Kicosia RF. Rat aorta-derived mural precursor cells express the Tie2 receptor an drepong directly to stimulation by angiopoietins. *J. Cell Sci.* 2003 116(17), 3635-43.

[11] Park YS, Kim NH and Jo I. Hypoxia and vascular endothelial growth factor acutely up-regulate angiopoietin-1 and Tie2 mRNA in bovine retinal pericytes. *Micorvas. Res.* 2003 65(2), 125-31.

[12] Tian S, Metheny-Barlow LJ, Hayes A and Li Ly. Direct action of Angiopietin-1 on mesenchymal cells: Stabilization of tumor neovasculature may contribute to tumor growth inhibition. *Proc. Am. Assoc. Cancer Res.* 2002 43, 500.

[13] Davis S, Aldrich TH, Jones PF, et. al. Isolation of angiopoietin-1, a ligand for the TIE2 receptor, by secretion-trap expression cloning. *Cell* 1996 87(7), 1161-9.

[14] Suri C, Jones PF, Patan S, et. al. Requisite role of angiopoietin-1, a ligand for the TIE2 receptor, during embryonic angiogenesis. *Cell* 1996 87(7), 1171-80.

[15] Maisonpierre PC, Suri C, Jones PC, et. Al. Angiopoietin-2, a natural antagonsit for Tie2 thaat disrupts in vivo angiogenesis. *Science* 1997 277(5322), 55-60.

[16] Hayes AJ, Huang WQ, MallahJ, Yang D, Leppman ME and Li LY. Angiooietin-1 and its receptor Tie2 participate in the refulation of capillary-like tubule formation and survival of endothelial cells. *Microvas. Res.* 1999 58(3), 224-37.

[17] Koblizek TI, Weiss C, Yancopoulos GD, Deutsch U and Risau W. Anfiopoietin-1 induces sprouting angiogenesis if vitro. *Curr. boil.* 1998 8(9), 529-32.

[18] Asahara T, Chen D, TakahashiT, et. al. Tie2 receptor lligands, angiopoietin-1 and angiopietin-2, modulate VEGF-ligand induced post natal neovascularization. *Circ. Res.* 1998 83(3), 233-40.

[19] Hawighorst T, Skobe M, Steit M, et. al. Activaiton of the tie2 receptor by angiooietin-1 enhances tumor vessel maturation and impairs squamous cell carcinoma growth. *Am. J. Path.* 2002 160(4), 1381-92.

[20] Lobov IB, Brooks PC and Lang RA. Angiopoietin-2 displays VEGF-dependent modulation of capillary structure and endothelial cell survival in vitro. *Proc. Natl. Acad. Sci. USA* 2002 99(17), 11205-10l

[21] Hatanaka H, Abe Y, Naruke M, et. al. Significant correlation between interleukin 10 expression and vascularization through angiopoietin/TIE2 networks in NSCLC. *Cancer Res.* 2001 7(5), 1287-92.

[22] Wong MP, Chan SY, Fu KH, et. al. The angiopoietins, tie2 and vascular endothelial growth factor are differentially expressed in the transformation os normal lung to NSCLC. *Lung Cancer* 2000 29(1), 11-22.

[23] Lord RV, Park JM, Wickramsinghe K, et. al. Vascualr endothelial growth factor and basic gibroblast growth factor expression in esophageal adenocarcinoma and Barret esophagus. *Gen. Thor. Surg.* 2003, 246-53.

[24] Obermair A, Kucera E, Mayerhofer K, et. Al. Vascular endothelial growth factor (VEGF) in human breast cancer : correlation with disease –free survival. *Int. J. Cancer* 1997 74, 455-8.

[25] O-charoenrat P, Rhys-Evans P and Eccles SA. Expression of vascular endothelial growth factor family members in head neck squamous cell carcinoma correlates with lymph node metastasis. *Cancer* 2001 92(3), 556-68.

[26] Fontanini G, Boldrini L, Chine S, Pisaturo F, Basolo F, Calcinai A, Lucchi M, Mussi A, Angeletti CA, Bevilacqua, G: Expression of vascular endothelial growth factor mRNA in non-small cell lung carcinomas. *Br. J. Cancer* 1999 79,363-369.

[27] Ohta Y, Endo Y, Tanaka M, Shimizu J, Oda M, Hayashi Y, Watanabe Y, Sasaki T: Significance of vascular endothelial growth factor messenger RNA expression in primary lung cancer. *Clin. Cancer Res.* 1996 2,1411-1416.

[28] Oshika Y, Nakamura M, Tojunaga T, et. Al. Expression of cell-associated isoform of vascular endothelial growth factor 189 and its prognostic relevance in NSCLC. *Int. J. Oncol.* 1998 12, 541-4.

[29] Volm M, Koomagi R, Mattern J: PD-ECGF, bFGF, and VEGF expression in non-small cell lung carcinomas and their association with lymph node metastasis. *Anticancer Res.* 1999 19,651-5.

[30] Shibusa T, Shijubo N, and Abe S: Tumor angiogenesis and vascular endothelial growth expression in stage I lung adenocarcinoma. *Clin. Cancer Res.* 1998 4,1483-1487.

[31] Shijubo N, Kojima H, Nagata M, Ohchi T, Suzuki A, Abe S and Sato N. Tumor angiogenesis of non-small cel lung cancer. *Microsc. Res. Tech.* 2003 60, 186-98.

[32] Merrick, DT, Haney, J, Petrunich, S, Sugita, M, Miller, YE, Keith, RL, Kennedy, TC and Franklin, WA. Overexpression of vascular endothelial growth factor and its receptors in brochial dysplasia demonstrated by quantitative RT-PCR analysis. *Lung* Cancer 2005 48,31-45.

[33] Keith RL, Miller YE, Gemmill RM, Drabkin HA, Dempsey EC, Haney J, LaRosa FG, Folkvord J, Kennedy TC, Prindiville S, Franklin WA: Angiogenic squamous dysplasia in bronchi of individuals at high risk for lung cancer. *Clin. Cancer Res.* 2000 6,1616-1625.

[34] Sugita M, Haney JL, Gemmill RM, Franklin WA: One-step duplex reverse transcription-polymerase chain reaction for quantitative assessment of RNA degradation. *Anal. Biochem*. 2001;295:113-6.

[35] Yoninaga Y, Mori A, Onodera H, Yasuda S, Oe H, Fujimoto A, Tachibana T and Imamura. Absence of smooth muscle actin-positive pericyte coverage of tumor vessels correaltes with hematogenous metastasis and prognosis of colorectal cancer patients. *Oncology* 2005 69(2), 159-66.

[36] Kakolyris S, Fox SB, Koukourakis M, Giatromanalaki A, Brown N, Leek RD, Leigh IM Gatter KC and Harris AL. Relationship of vascular maturationin breast cancer blood vessels to vascular density and metastasis, assessed by expression of a novel basement membrane component, LH39. *Br. J. Cancer* 2000 82(4), 844-51.

[37] Frost JK, Ball WC Jr, Levin ML, Tockman MS, Erozan YS, Fupta K, Eggleston JC, Pressman NJ, Donithan MP, Kimball AW: Sputum cytopathology: use and potential in monitoring the workplace environment by screening for biological effects of exposure. *J. Occup. Med.* 1986 28,692-703.

[38] Venman BJW, van Boxem TJM, Smit EF, Postmus PE, Sutedja TG: Outcome of bronchial carcinoma in situ. *Chest* 2000 117,1572-6.

[39] Bota S, Auliac J-B, Paris C, et. al. Follow-up of bronchial precancerous lesions and carcinoma *in situ* using fluorescence endoscopy. *Am. J. Respir. Crit. Care Med.* 2001 164,1688-1693.

[40] Soufla F, Sifakis S, Baritaki S, Zafiropoulos A, Koumantakis E and Apandidos DA. VEGF, FGF2, TGFB1 and TGFBR1 mRNA expression levels correlate with the malignant transformation of the uterine cervix. *Cancer Lett.* 2005 221(1), 105-18.

[41] Denhart BC, Guidi AJ, Tognazzi K, Dvorak and Brown LF. Vascular permeability factor/vascular endothelial growth factor and its receptors in oral and laryngeal squamous cell carcinoma and dysplasia. *Lab. Invest.* 1997 77(6), 659-64.

[42] Brennan PA, Umar T, Wilson AW and Mellor TK. Expression of type 2 nitric oxide synthase and vascular endothelial growth factor in oral dysplasia. *J. Oral Maxillofac. Surg.* 2002 60(12), 1455-60.

[43] Obermair A, Bancher-Todesca D, Bilgi S, Kaider A, Kohlberger P, Mullauer-Ertl S, Leodolter S and Gitsch G. Correlation of vascular endothelial growth factor expression and microvessel density in cervical intraepithelial neoplasia. *J. Natl. Cancer Inst.* 89:1212-7, 1997.

[44] Isaka S, Sawai K, Tomiie M, Kamiura S, Koyama M, Azuma C, Ishiguro S, Murata Y and Saji F. Expression of platelet-derived endothelial cell growth factor/thymidine phosphorylase in cervical intraepithelial neoplasia. *Int. J. Oncol.* 2002 21(2), 281-7.

[45] Chang YS, Munn LL, Hillsley MV, et.al. Effect of vascular endothelial growth factor on cultured cell monolayer transport properties. *Microvasc. Res.* 2000 59,265-77.

[46] Bates Do. The chronic effect of vascular endothelial growth factor on individually perfused frog mesenteric microvessels. *J. Physiol.* 1998 513, 308-22.

[47] Mironchik Y, Winnard PT, Vesuna F, et. Al. Twist overexpression induces in vivo angiogenesis and correlates with chromosomal instability in breast cancer. *Cancer Res.* 2005 65(23), 10801-9.

In: Dysplasia
Editors: L. M. Sexton and H. J. Leach
ISBN 978-1-61942-600-9


*Chapter VII*

# SUDDEN CARDIAC DEATH SYNDROME - ARRHYTHMOGENIC RIGHT VENTRICULAR DYSPLASIA/CARDIOMYOPATHY AS MOST FREQUENT CAUSE OF FATAL ARRHYTHMIAS

***Ivana I. Vranic[1,*] and Tijana Simic[2]***
[1]University Institute for cardiovascular diseases, Clinical Center of Serbia, Serbia
[2]University Institute for anesthesiology and rescucitation, Clinical Center of Serbia, Serbia

## ABSTRACT

In the United States 350,000 people die yearly of SCD which does not spare any age, gender, or socioeconomic group. Major cause of SCD accounts for CAD, but smaller percentage is due to cardiac diseases other then CAD. The main substrate of latter are cardiac arrhythmias, mainly caused by ARVD/C, Long QT sy and WPW sy in those otherwise healthy population. Special problem exists in professional sports and dieing during sport activities, in spite being regularly thoroughly examined.

The most mysterious among aforementioned is arrhythogenic right ventricular dysplasia and/or cardiomyopathy (21 clinical genotype types) which unfortunately, apparently, has no clinical warning sign at the early

* E mail: ivvra@beotel.yu; Koste Todorovica 8; 11 000 Belgrade; Serbia, Europe.

stage, sometimes having SCD for the first and only presenting dramatic event. The arrhythmias leading to SCD may be identified by electrophysiological testing, and significant percentage of patients can have polymorphic VT or VF as the only inducible arrhythmia, which seems to be the exact scenario for fatal outcome in the whole group of patients. So what might be the underlying cause and could it be prevented?

ARVD/C is genetically inherited condition with autosomal-dominant pattern of inheritance (as most common), as consequence of single gene mutations witch lead to complex patterns of altered localization of desmosomal proteins. These mutations may change cytosolic pools of cell-cell junction proteins which lead to desmosome disorganization and gap junction distortion. Latter is explanation for loss of contact between cardiomyocites and earlier start of apoptosis.

Pathological hallmark of ARVD/C is the atrophy of myocites with fatty or fibro-fatty infiltration of the right ventricle. Typical clinical picture encompasses arrhythmias with left bundle branch block morphology and ventricular tachyarrhythmias, while less frequent presentation are signs of right heart failure (fatigue and shortness of breath). Disease may be localized or widespread, with biventricular involvement in some cases.

Valid WHO criteria during last 12 years failed to detect disease at its early stage and recommended diagnostic methods were shown to have low sensitivity for majority of patients even in its overt phase (because of lack of scoring system). Investigation of this population is further complicated by disease rarity and lack of large databases. New research published data give priority to vectorcardiography and ultrasound.

The possible explanation for this lies in the existence of specific place in the heart exposed to most physical forces during cardiac cycle. Nevertheless, this place is *locus minoris rezistentio* during contraction and relaxation of the heart. It is presently focus of ongoing clinical study regarding two aforementioned methods in detecting early stage of ARVD/C. It is also registered by WIPO as SOPHIE methodology (suggesting wisdom to detect). Soon enough we can expect this technique to be incorporated in newly medical equipment (for stratification of risk for SCD).

## Background

Sudden cardiac death is no respecter of geographic boundaries and it continues to represent an important challenge because of major difficulties in identifying those individuals at risk and in responding to timely prevention from catastrophic event.

The mode and time of SCD are unexpected, which is a generally accepted definition for death heralded by abrupt loss of consciousness within an hour of the onset of acute symptoms. Clinical, scientific, medico-legal and social issues must be considered to fully reach definition for SCD: prodromes, onset, cardiac arrest, and progression to biological death [1].

## Incidence

The incidence of SCD is approximately 300 000- 350 000 annually which accounts for an incidence 0,1-0,2% per year among the population >35years of age. The overall incidence is 1 to 2 / 1000. Various estimates suggest that at least two-thirds of all SCDs occur due to coronary heart disease as a first clinical event or among subgroups of pts thought to be at a relatively low risk for SCD [2,3].

## Circadyal Rhythm

Circadyal rhythm analysis derives definite diurnal, weekly and seasonal pattern. Throughout the day, peak incidence happens during the early morning hours, and through the night soon after midnight [4]. This phenomena can be explained by hormonal disbalance in their prevalence: adrenalin/noradrenalin steep rise in the morning and prolactin peak during the night. Nevertheless, it might point to susceptibility of electrical conduction delay to hormone stimulation and activity of sympatico-parasympatetic ascendancy. In a 7 days of a week it is stress activated Monday syndrome obviously derived by sympathetic activity, and weekends off stress nivelation by natural antioxydative substances like prostacyclin and adenosine (endothelial derived preservation parahormones). Seasonal pattern is preponderant to winter months because of usual low temperatures in the northern hemisphere, and also of the Moon and Sun influence during the year.

## Age

There are two ages of clusterring registered for SCD: between birth and 6 months of age (the sudden infant death syndrome) due to concealed congenital heart disease like Uhl's anomaly, and between 45 and 75 years of age, due to CAD and ARVD. The incidence of SCD is 100-fold less in adolescents and adults below 30 years of age, than in adults above 35[5].

# ETIOLOGY: GENETICS, MUTATIONS, DESMOSOMAL CYTOSOLIC CHANGES

ARVD/C is genetically inherited condition with autosomal-dominant pattern of inheritance (as most common), as consequence of single gene mutations witch lead to complex patterns of altered localization of desmosomal proteins. The linkage analysis in the ARVD affected families focused on chromosome 14 and located the ARVD gene in the proximity of D14S42 locus 14q23-q24 [6]. That region includes genes for beta-spectrin and for alpha-actinin.The existing hypothesis confirmed the possibility of mutation in that region to be involved in pathogenesis of ARVD, by assumption that functionally related genes are often located on the same chromosome.

The degeneration of skeletal muscle seen in Duchenne/Becker muscular dystrophy, similar to process in cardiomyocites in ARVD, and structural similarities between alpha-actinin and N-terminal domain of dystrophin, postulated another possibility, the involvement of alpha –actinin gene mutation in ARVD patients [7]. However, published research data found alpha -actinin molecule in different isoforms, which led to conclusion that mutation on the specific gene does not cause functional alteration in all isoforms.

Recently, more attention was payed to the well known clinical fact of right ventricular early involvement in Becker's dystrophy. Precisely, the right ventricle undergoes maximal streching of myocardial tissue during cardiac cycle and published data confirmed that dystrophin complex was related to stretch/modulated calcium channel in sarcolaema [8]. The possible explanation implied with intense stretching of myocardial fibers thus having an impact on stretch/modulated calcium channels in membrane and affecting dystrophin complex intracellulary. By analogy with right ventricular invovment in Becker`s dystrophy ARVD was found to be with similar scenario as having a product of ARVD gene to be component of dystrophin complex.

Synchronous propagation of electrical current in cardiomyocites is highly dependent on number and spatial distribution of gap junction channels,the only place in membrane where transfer of depolarizing current can occur. These membrane areas with maximal possible amount of proteins in lipid bilyer are thus rigid and susceptible to fragmentation in response to shear stress of

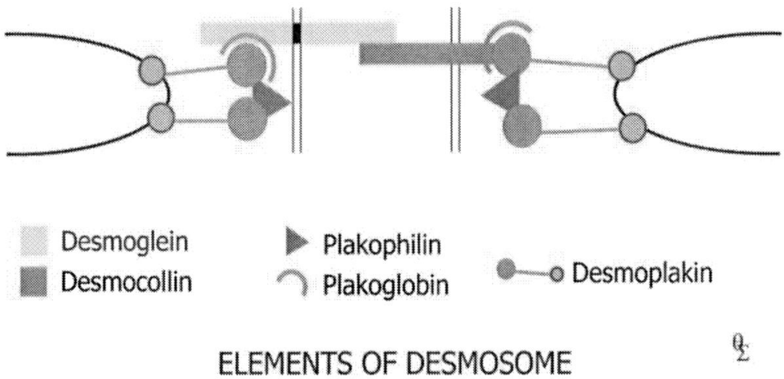


Figure 1. Schematic view of desmosome components.

contracting ventricular myocardium.Concerning physiology, it is of uttermost importance to secure areas of gap junctions by developing cell to cell adhesion junctions that stabilixe sarcolemma. Gap junctions are dependent on structure and function of adhesion junctions specially in the cardiomyocites.

It was postulated that extent of electrical coupling at gap junctions is determined by the extent of mechanical coupling i.e. cell to cell adhesion junctions in cardiac myocites.

Both mechanical junctions responsible for intercellular adhesion of cardiomyocites (fascia adherens junctions and desmosomes) consist of three components: adhesion molecules, linker proteins and citoscletal proteins.

Genetic defect in expression of one of these components cause an abnormal linkage between mechanical junctions and cytoskeleton progressively remodeling the myocite gap junctions at intercalated discs135

, thus compromiting normal conduction and creating a highly arrhythmogenic substrate. Good example is Naxos disease where mutation of the gene responsible for encoding plakoglobin, intercellular linkage protein and component of desmosome, leads to remodeling of cardiomyocite gap junctions and disruption of membrane leads to mechanical and electrical mismatch in like manner leading to arrhytmogenesis and enhancing the risc for SCD.

There are two distinctive disease mechanisms in the cell-cell junction cardiomyopathies that could be descriebed with certainity: first, mechanical, that explains discontinuities between cytoskeleton because of the abnormal adhesion of desmosomal proteins; and second nuclear signaling hypothesis that finds deficit of γ-catenin (plakoglobin) and β-catenin that contribute to disease pathogenesis. Above mentioned mutations may change cytosolic pools of cell-cell junction proteins which may lead to desmosome disorganization and gap junction distortion. Latter is explanation for loss of contact between cardiomyocites and earlier start of apoptosis. If the desmosomes are disorganized the gap junctions should be distorted. Gap junctions are playing a role in electrical coupling of cardiomyopathies which may explain slow conduction. Specific patterns of altered localization of cell-cell junction proteins correlate with disease phenotypes and 21 clinical forms of ARVD/C [9].

## Apoptosis in the Heart

Morphogenesis and remodeling during heart development involve coordinated regulation of cell proliferation and apoptosis. Apoptosis, or programmed cell death, undergoes a characteristic cascade of biochemical events in which specific membrane phospholipids are exposed to cleavage of specific caspase enzymes. In the heart, clear evidence points toward focal apoptosis as a contributor to development of the embryonic outflow tract, cardiac valves, conducting system, and the developing coronary vasculature [10]. Much has been discovered about the molecular control of apoptosis since its initial description as a series of morphological events, that play a critical role in heart formation, such as formation of septa between cardiac chambers and valves[11].

The adult cardiomyocite has limited (if any) ability to proliferate. Correspondingly, apoptosis is observed infrequently in adult hearts. The finding that cardiomyocyte apoptosis occurs in the end stage human heart indicates that mechanical stretch with volume overload and raised ventricular end diastolic pressure as well as catecholamine stimulation are trigger factors in those patients. On the other side, high levels of apoptosis have been observed in arrhythmogenic right ventricular dysplasia, a condition characterized by myocardial replacement with fibro fatty material[12].

The recent results publicated by Dr Jeff Safitz clearly demonstrate that pts with ARVD are 10fold more susceptible to mechanical stretch and electrical force then normal cardiomyocites, explaining why those pts are at risk for early and massive apoptosis.

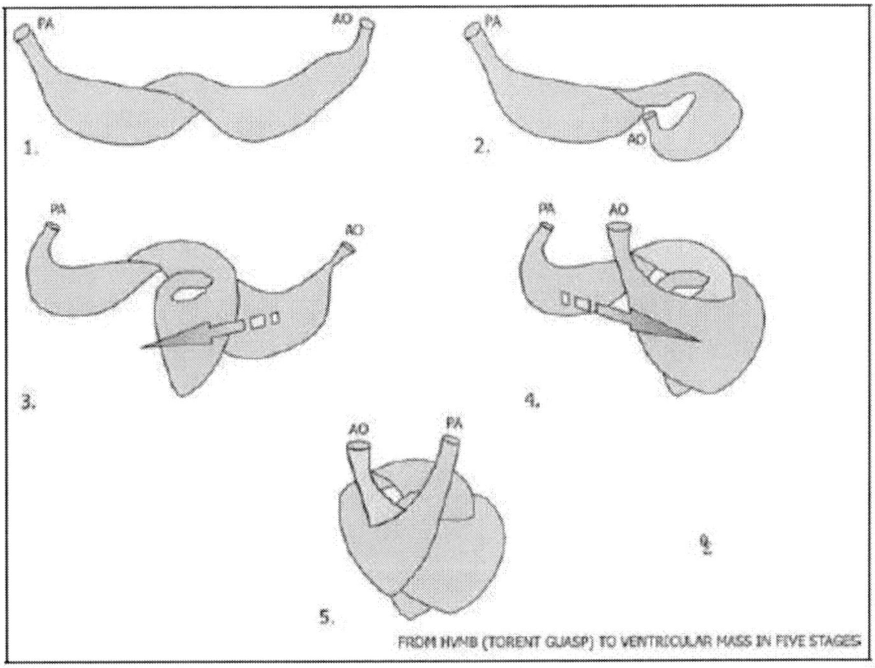


Figure 2. Simplified explaination of heart's development morphological changes.

## PATHOANATOMICAL AND PATHOPHISIOLOGICAL BASIS OF THE DISEASE

During embriological development human heart follows ontogenetical transformations and repeating the pattern of the Universe it finally becomes double helix[13]. According to Torrent-Guasp's model human heart is double helicoid struucture organized by singular muscular band [14,15,16], (Fig 1).

Specific place in the human ventricular muscular band (HVMB) is the knot formed by twisting along the instrinsic axis and folding for up to 180 degreees[17,18]. That central twist of HVMB, or knot defines two loops: basal, from pulmonary artery root to the central fold and apical loop, from central fold to the aortic root [19,20], (Fig 2).

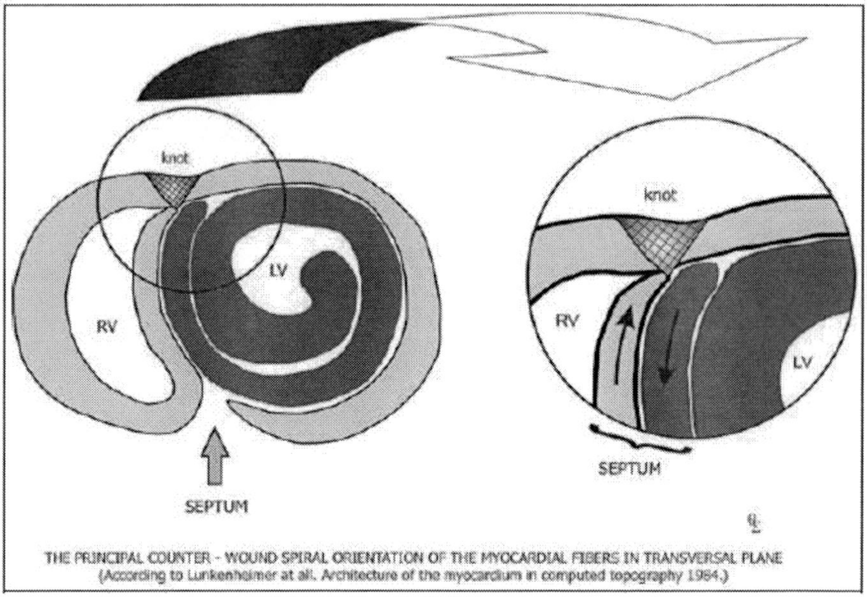


Figure 3. Arrows represent different vectors of force of contraction through LV systole "vide intra".

The parts of basal loop are free right ventricular wall and left free ventricular wall divided by posterior linear border of right ventricular cavity (sulcus inerventricularis posterior)[13,18]. The fibers forming apical loop after the knot make descendent part and with 90 degrees turn propagate upwards as ascending part to the root of the aorta.(Fig 1)

During the cardiac cycle the wave of excitation goes along ventricular muscular band and contraction follows the same route[14,15,16]. The cardiac cycle thus, is the consequence of spatial orientation of VMB and net effect of forces developed inside some [17]. The heart movements trough normal cardiac cycle to our impression resemble the rhythm of Cuban salsa: ejection, twist-untwist, suction.

One of the first signs in the early stage of ARVD is the abnormal movement of basal part of the interventricular septum, seen by TDI on 2D echo, already described and named "V sign" by Dr Ivana Vranic few years ago, now transparent to understanding with pathoanatomical interplay of HVMB and early apoptotic process due to mechanical streching in the specific point of septum interventricularis named "$\tau$" point [21], (Fig 3,4).

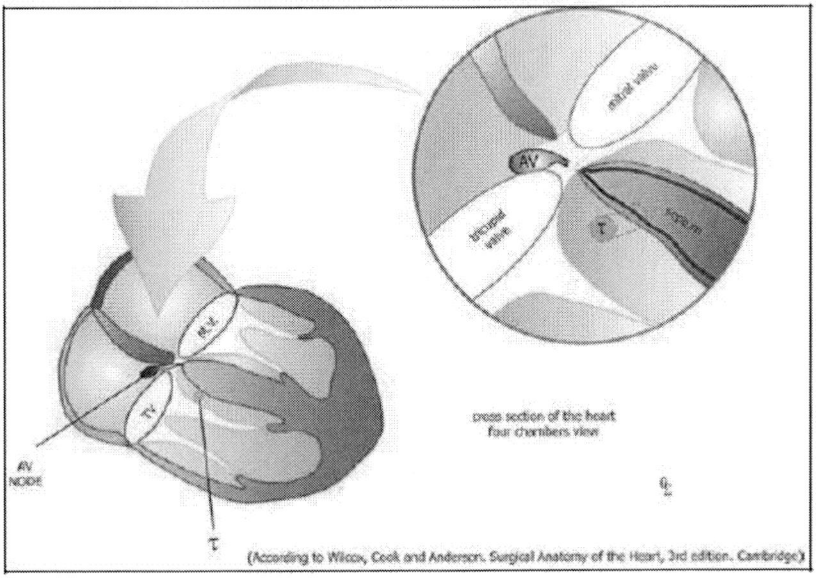


Figure 4. Location of the "τ" point.

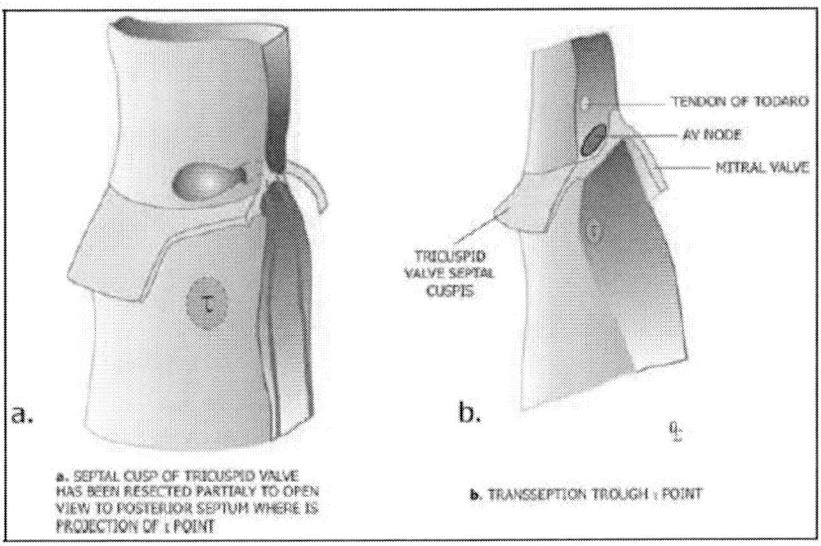


Figure 5. Location of the "τ" point.

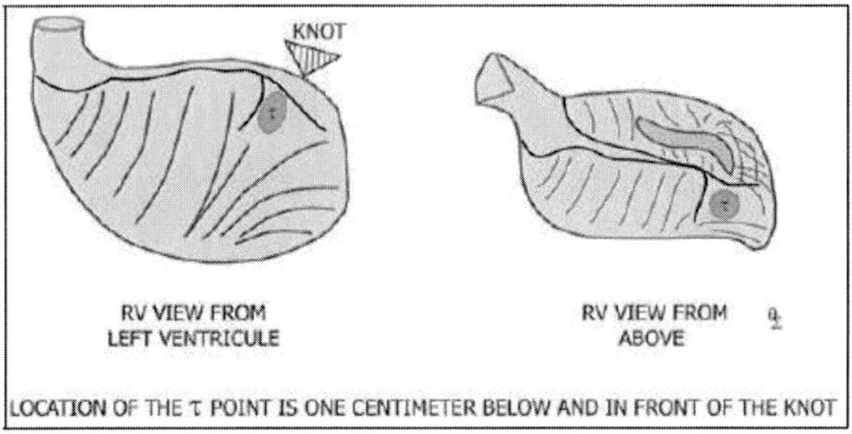


Figure 6. Knot is proximal to the "τ" point.

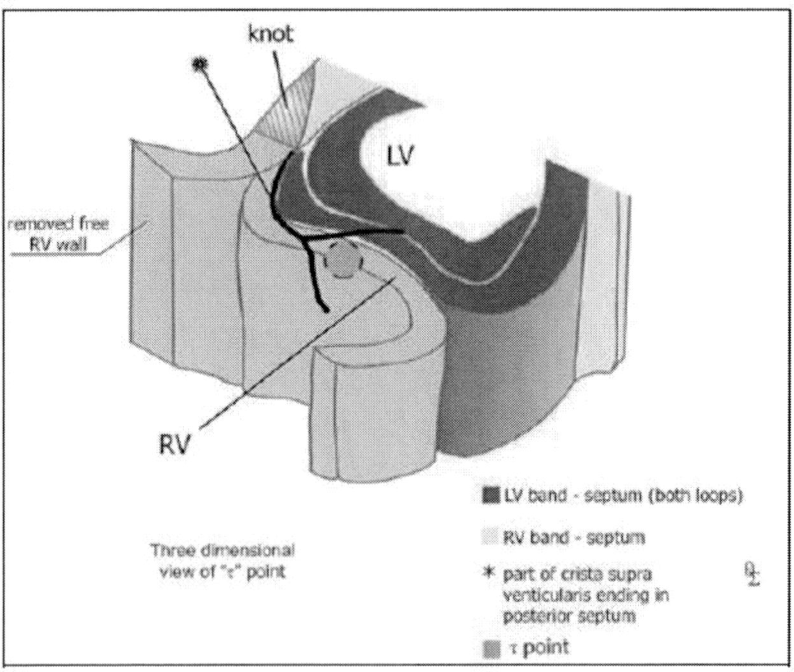


Figure 7. Transsection of IVS at the level of knot.

Tau point and knot of MVB are very close to each other and connecting fibers exist from knot to right ventricular band-septal portion as well as to the LV first loop and LV second loop.

Thus structure of septum is of a special interest concerning impact of statical forces implyed in ARVD. According to Torrent-Guasp model of the heart, both ventricles participate in formation of septum. Right ventricle with anterior and posterior reccurent fibres, a tiny superfitial fibers that have vertical direction. Deeper there is a layer of ascendent segment fibers ,that after sinking into the anterior interventicular sulcus, run obliquely and upwads in the destianation of aortic root. Third fiber direction in septum belongs to the descending segment whose orientation is different and at 90 degrees crossis the former layer. This is also clearly visible on the histological preparations of septum (Fig 2, Fig 6).

Note the existence of two patterns of myofibrillar space orientation in ventricular septum:a longitudinal, belonging to right ventricular band and transversal, belonging to left ventricular band (Fig 7).

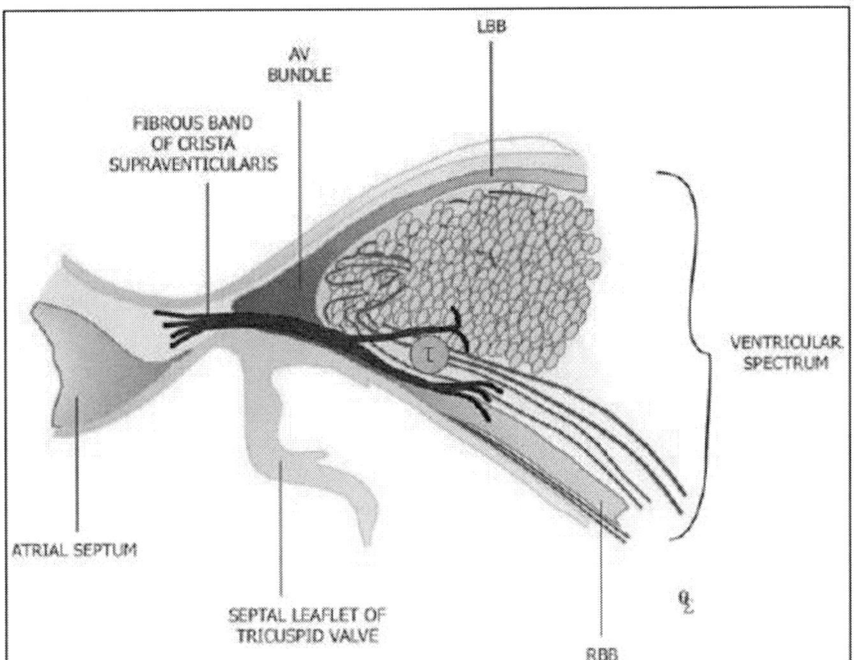


Figure 8. Schematic hystological architecture of interventricular septum with regard to fibrous anchoring of CSV and Tau point.

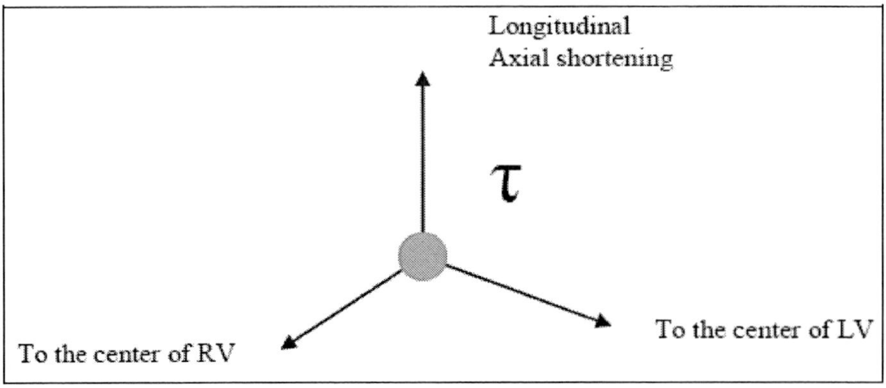


Figure 9. Schematic representation of different traction forces at the "τ" point.

Crista supraventicularis is finishing by deep anchoring in posterior septum approximatelly 1 cm bellow the knot divided in two parts:one part ending in the internal loop of LV and the other one in the septal part of exterior LV loop and right ventricle (Fig 6,7).

Tau point is located directly between these two parts exposed to three different tracton forces which stretch along projections in three ortogonal system (Fig 8).

First force is centripetal, e.i to the centre of LV and is a consequence of the first loop contraction. Second force is a consequence of propagation of electromechanical wave along the muscular band making the two layers of septum to move in opposite directions from the "τ" point (Fig 2). Third force is active in saggital plane, and is a consequence of ejection phase due to the action of longitudinal forces along the heart axis.

Myocardium at that point undergoes maximum shear stress trough cardiac cycle and in special pathological conditions is first to degenerate.

There is no other point along myocardial band that undergoes traction of more physical forces, so it represents "locus resistentiae minoris" for adiposis prone patients. At that particular point of the heart, "τ" point starts beginning of loss of heart SALSA rhythm and deteriorization seen as sudden jerking movements. At that point, begins forming of an obstacle for normal electrical conduction and cause for instability and fatal arrhythmias.

# DEFINITION

Right ventricular dysplasia/cardiomyopathy is genetically transmitted condition characterized by structural and functional abnormalities that involve mostly the right ventricle and sometimes the left ventricle as well. It is caused by the replacement of myocardial tissue by fat and fibrous tissue. The most striking morphological feature of the disease is massive diffuse or segmental loss of myocardium and replacement with fat and fibrous tissue in the mediomural and epicardial layers of the right ventricular free wall[22,23].

## Clinical Forms and Genetics. Classification of Right Ventricular Cardiomyopathies

Dr Guy Fontaine[24] has proposed new classification of ARVC during the last SCD Internet symposium wich encompassed folowing similar conditions:

### *ARVD*

***Phenotype*:** This disease is, as is with most of the other forms of ARVC, an inherited condition transmitted in a dominant form with variable expressions and penetrance in family members (20 to 50%). It is generally discovered during adolescence by signs of ventricular arrhythmias originating in the right ventricle. Sudden death can be the first presenting symptom especially during endurance and competitive sports. It is generally a progressive condition, but the disease may remain stable for decades.

***Histology*:** The epicardial and frequently mediomural layers of RV myocardium are occupied by fat and fibrosis. Some aspects suggest that the pathologic process starts in the mediomural layers mostly extending toward the epicardium, which can be totally made of fat and fibrosis, wrongly suggesting that the disease progresses from epicardium to endocardium. Fibrosis generally borders or embeds surviving fibers. Full thickness of the RV myocardium is necessary to depict the typical topographic features of the lesions. Therefore, histology is the gold standard to ascertain the diagnosis. The frust forms and forms observed at the beginning of the disease, especially those observed in family members, can be difficult to diagnose. Involvement of the left ventricle is frequently observed mostly at the apex, which looks covered by fat. However, some focal zones of fibrosis and fatty tissue can be found all over the full thickness of LV myocardium. This may explain the decrease in the LV function found even in the moderate forms of the disease.

***Genotype:*** Genes identified are coding for Desmoplakin and recently Plakophilin 2 and Desmoglein 2. These genes are parts of the desmosomal structure and fascia adherens, which plays a major role in longitudinal cell-cell adhesion. However, Transforming Growth Factor (TGF Beta3) is a new gene related to the phenotypic presentation of one of these cardiomyopathies. Plakophillin 2 appears currently as the most frequently observed gene (11 to 43% of the series).

### *Biventricular Dysplasia*

***Phenotype*:** Because of the loss of myocardial tissue of the left ventricle, this form frequently leads to congestive heart failure.

***Histology:*** In this form, the same evidence of fatty tissue and fibrosis is observed in both ventricles. However, the disease seems to progress from epicardium to endocardium as opposed to classical ARVD, where fibrosis and fat seems to start in the mediomural layers.

### *RVD without Arrhythmia Quiescent*

***Phenotype:*** There are no obvious arrhythmias as opposed to the previous form. This might be related to the fact that the arrhythmogenic substrate is totally silent or that minor arrhythmias are present, but not severe enough to lead to hospitalization.

***Histology:*** In this form, observed in 3.7% of the general population, the typical histologic pattern of ARVD is observed in the RV free wall. However, the arrhythmogenic substrate is dormant. It is postulated that the occurrence of arrhythmias that may lead to sudden death is either due to the development of critical electrophysiologic parameters leading to sustained re-entry or the result of neutrophiles activation or both.

### *RVD with Congestive Heart Failure*

***Phenotype:*** This can be the result of two different mechanisms. The first is due to major progression of the dysplastic phenomenon, producing more and more myocardium by fat and fibrosis in the right ventricle, and leading to subsequent involvement of the left ventricle by the same disease process. The second is due to a superimposed myocarditis (see below). Because of absence or minor arrhythmias, these cases can mimic Idiopathic dilated cardiomyopathy.

***ARVD + Superimposed Myocarditis***

Clinical as well as histologic data, may exhibit various forms of myocarditis superimposed on ARVD suggesting a particular susceptibility of dysplastic myocardium to inflammatory phenomena in particular viruses (this concept can be extended to other forms of cardiomyopathies). The presence of coxsackies as well as adenoviruses has been observed in the myocardium of ARVD patients. In most cases myocarditis involves both the right and left ventricle. Both the severity of left ventricular involvement and speed of myocarditis progression, determines the prognosis. Clinical patterns are quite variable.

***Quiescent***

***Phenotype***: Asymptomatic.

***Histology***: presence of lymphocytes is common (0.1-5.5%) in the general population. In our opinion it seems nevertheless more frequent in ARVD patients.

***Hyper Acute***

***Phenotype:*** Fever, asthenia, dyspnea, hypotension, fulminant heart failure and death within a few days.

***Histology:*** Diffuse round cells infiltration, polymorphonuclear, eosinophils.

***Acute***

***Phenotype:*** Fever, Chest pain, AV conduction disorder. May last from a few days up to several weeks and is associated with the release of cardiac enzymes (troponine).

***Histology:*** Round cells (lymphocytes). Value of endocardial biopsies that may lead to therapeutic implications (Beta-interferon).

***Chronic***

***Phenotype:*** Moderate clinical signs of heart failure, asthenia, dyspnea, etc.

***Histology:*** Healed myocarditis leaves patchy areas of "replacement" fibrosis.

Lymphocytes have disappeared or remain in small quantities.

***Chronic-active***

***Phenotype:*** Moderate clinical signs of heart failure, asthenia, dyspnea, increasing with time, palpitations, syncope, etc.

***Histology:*** Myocarditis, which is frequently multifocal, progresses replacing more and more myocardium by fibrosis and patchy zones of adipocytes. Lymphocytes are present. These multiple forms explain the polymorphism of clinical presentations. We think that superimposed myocarditis is a major cause of the trigger of arrhythmias and sudden death.Therefore the pathology of the hearts of patients who died suddenly have shown more frequently than in the common forms of RVD the evidence of signs of inflammation. Gene mutations explaining viral susceptibility is an open question.

***Naxos Disease***

This is a very rare disease discovered in the island of Naxos (Greece) in 24 patients from 6 families. The form of transmission is recessive; some other isolated cases have been discovered in the world.

***Phenotype*:** The phenotype is identical to classical ARVD associated with Woolly hair

and Keratoderma.

***Histology*:** Typical ARVD association. The association of signs

of myocarditis and arrhythmias is frequent, as is sudden death.

***Genotype*:** Plakoglobin truncation is the monogenic factor producing the disease. All patients are homozygous. The asymptomatic heterozygous patients may have Right Ventricular Outflow Tract ventricular tachycardia.

***Israelian Desmoplakin Recessive Dysplasia***

***Phenotype*:** There is a syndrome found in the non-Jewish population of Israel associated with woolly hair, keratoderma and RVD similar to Naxos disease.

***Genotype*:** Desmoplakin truncation is the monogenic factor producing the disease.

***Venetian Desmoplakin Dominant Dysplasia: Transmission is Autosomal Dominant***

***Phenotype*:** Seems similar to ARVD.

***Histology*:** Similar to ARVD.

***Genotype*:** Desmoplakine located in series between plakoglobin and desmin, supporting the complex actin-myosin, is responsible for the disease.

***Uhl's Anomaly: A Rare Anomaly***

***Phenotype*:** Two forms.

Pediatric form: Newborns (differential diagnosis with Ebstein disease) with congestive heart failure.

Adult form: Arrhythmias, congestive heart failure or both. This form is frequently confused with ARVD.

***Histology***: The pathologic examination is pathognomonic and unmistakable. There is total absence of myocardium on the RV free wall consisting only of epicardium and endocardium separated by a thin layer of adipocytes occupied by coronary vessels, which could exhibit abnormal proliferation of the media. Thus, the wall is, properly speaking, transparent.

### *ARVD Mimicking Uhl's Anomaly*

***Phenotype***: One case with huge RV (Dr G Fontaine). Extremely thin RV free wall mimicking Uhl's anomaly (all imaging techniques).

***Histology:*** After heart transplant for terminal heart failure, a thin layer of myocardium was present. The wall was translucent but not transparent. This is therefore different from typical Uhl's anomaly.

### *Biventricular Spongy Dysplasia*

***Phenotype***: Slowly progressing congestive heart failure. One case from Portugal (Dr G Fontaine). No other case in the literature.

***Histology***: Total disappearance of myocardium in RV with thick endocardium and epicardium. LV dissociated by interstitial fat with minor fibrosis, suggesting apoptosis.

### *Catecholaminergic VTs*

***Phenotype:*** Episodes of Polymorphic VTs triggered by effort or psychological stress. High risk of sudden death.

***Histology:*** Two presentations:

*With structural heart disease:* Histology similar to classical ARVD.

*Without structural heart disease.*

***Genotype***: Mutation of the gene coding for RyR2 Ryanodine receptor on Sarcoplasmic reticulum playing a role in the regulation of intracellular calcium. The overload of calcium can explain the particular morphology of ventricular arrhythmias. This is different from ARVD arrhythmias, which are mostly the result of slow intramyocardial conduction and reentry.

### *Brugada Syndrome (BS) (Some Patients Only)*

***Phenotype:*** Nocturnal sudden death, dizziness, “vasovagal syncope”. In some cases this syndrome shows an overlapping pattern with ARVD.

Nevertheless, effectiveness of Isoprenaline in the BS is in sharp contrast with ARVD, where it is used to induce ventricular arrhythmias. Therefore, it seems appropriate to include in the database only those BS ECG patients who meet the new ARVD criteria.

***Histology***: Pathology of some cases of BS who died suddenly showed, in 38% of them, structural heart disease, some with signs of inflammation/fibrosis andothers with a typical histologic pattern of ARVD.

***Genotype***: Multiple mutations in SCN5A that now appears as a cofactor rather than the unique cause of the disease.

***Right Ventricular Outflow Tract (RVOT) (about 50% of Patients)***

***Phenotype***: Extrasystoles, runs of repetitive short runs of ventricular tachycardia. Imaging techniques have identified a structural heart disease.

***Histology***: A typical pattern of dysplasia localized to the infundibular area has been reported (including small vessels disease).

***Septal Ventricular Outflow Tract (SVOT)***

Ventricular extrasystoles progressing to VT have been observed in intraseptal exploration by using a special needle probe inserted inside the RV septum during surgery and showing highly fragmented potentials.

***Left Ventricular Outflow Tract (LVOT)***

Extrasystoles and VTs have been recently identified. Structural heart disease has not been reported yet.

***Fat Dissociation Syndrome (FDS)***

***Phenotype***: No symptoms, presence of hypersignal of fat at MRI examination (false positive diagnosis for ARVD). The risk of sudden death is very low.

***Histology***: Presence of fatty tissue in the right ventricular myocardium has been known by pathologists for a long time. However, its quantitative assessment is recent. In addition, fat in the RV appears to be specific to the human species. This is observed in up to 60% of the general population. It has not been observed in the RV of eight non-Bonobo monkeys. Therefore, FDS seems to be the result of a mutation that has occurred specifically in the human species. Basically, there is no fibrosis in FDS, which seems less dangerous than ARVD.

## Clinical Picture

ARVD manifests by means of a wide spectrum of clinical presentations, including mechanical myocardial dysfunction and various arrhythmias, generally of right ventricular origin, such as isolated extrasystoles, nonsustained or sustained ventricular tachycardia (VT), and ventricular fibrillation responsible for SD. Atrial arrhythmias are sometimes present because of dilated right atrium.

## Diagnosis

Diagnosis of ARVD is based on the presence of major and minor criteria encompassing structural, electrocardiographic, arrhythmic, and genetic factors. Among these criteria inverted T waves beyond V1 are a sign of diagnostic value that should attract attention, particularly in young patient with a normal heart at physical examination. However, these criteria are about to be reconsidered on more objective grounds.

The recognition of mild, fruste, or localized forms of the disease remains a clinical challenge. It is difficult to diagnose ARVD in patients with minimal right ventricular abnormalities by echocardiographic or contrast angiographic examination. Magnetic resonance imaging is a promising technique in showing right ventricular anatomy and function as well as in characterizing the composition of the right ventricular wall, especially with regard to the presence of adipose tissue.

## Pitfalls in Diagnosing ARVD

Arrhythmogenic right ventricular dysplasia is a genetic disorder followed by peculiar RV involvement and its structural and functional abnormalities (due to the replacement of myocardium by fatty and fibrous tissues) and electrical instability that precipitates ventricular arrhythmias and sudden death. However, all non-invasive and invasive methods of evaluating RV structure and function have inherent limitations, which are due to the complex anatomy of RV. Evaluation of the RV can present awesome experience since of its very complicated geometry and fact of being separated into three parts: inflow, outflow and belonging body which is crescentic and truncated. Not to mention the right ventricular free wall which also has a variable trabecular pattern that in combination with its retrosternal position limits precise measurement of cavity size and wall thickness. Nevertheless, tricuspid anterior plane systolic excursion (TAPSE) has been shown to correlate with its overall function (in adults), particularly in systole, as assessed by ejection fraction, which can be objectively estimated by radionuclide ventriculography (done in a standard way). The recognition of mild, *fruste*, or localized forms of the disease remains a clinical challenge. It is difficult to diagnose ARVD in patients with minimal right ventricular abnormalities by echo or contrast angiography examination. So far only V sign has been attributed as pathognomonic in ARVD but no other signs have been reported yet. Standardized diagnostic criteria have been proposed by the ISFC, however this condition may be overlooked by the insufficiency of its signs at the early stage of disease.

## Relevance of Right Ventricular Function

The right ventricle is a structurally and functionally complex chamber whose importance has been neglected previously. However, it maintains haemodynamic stability by propelling systemic venous blood returning from the right atrium through the pulmonary vascular bed. Therefore, right ventricular dysfunction is relevant in a variety of conditions such as: chronic lung disease, primary pulmonary vascular disease, pulmonary thrombo-embolic disease, myocardial infarction, congenital heart disease and cardiopulmonary transplantation. Right ventricular diastolic function is first to be affected in those conditions with relative preservation of systolic function. Nevertheless, in ARVD patients diastolic function may be pseudonormalized (due to the phenomenon of ventricular interdependence) in the clinically silent form of the disease and having only slightly impaired systolic function of a right ventricle.

## Echocardiography in Diagnosing ARVD

In the former sugessted protocol for ARVC search by echo, it was highlighted that thorough and systematic examination of both ventricles should be performed and particularly because of the fact that the disease process can be localised also in the left ventricle. The procedure must be reproducible and relevant in the context of a clinical setting. Therefore, the suggested protocol concentrated on the sites of disease predilection, namely the RV apex, inflow and outflow tracts- the so-called “triangle of dysplasia”. The degree of RV dilatation can be described in relation to the left ventricle (LV) with RV enlargement described as follows: mild: RV enlarged but a 2D area less than LV area; moderate: RV area equals LV area; severe: RV larger than LV area.

## Dimensions of Right Ventricle Region of Interest

Foale et al studied normal adult right ventricles to determine the reproducibility of various tomographic planes and to obtain measurements of normal cavity sizes. From this study the most easily obtained and reproducible measurements were ascertained and are suggested as part of the standard examination. Because the inflow tract (RVIT), ventricular body, and outflow tract (RVOT) are three distinct regions of the right ventricle that are orientated in different axis, two measurements of each region should be obtained from separate views: RVIT1 and RVIT3, RVOT1 and RVOT3, and RVSAX (short-axis) and RVLAX (long-axis)

Typically the echocardiogram is performed with the subject in the left lateral decubitus position. At least three sinus beats of each view should be recorded during quiet respiration or at end expiration. If the patient is in atrial fibrillation at least 5 beats should be recorded.

For each view, the gain and compression should be optimized so that the best echocardiographic image of the endocardial borders is obtained. The selection of harmonics or fundamental frequency should depend upon which yields the best definition of structures. The depth should be selected that allows visualization of all of the structures of interest. All images should have an ECG tracing and clear calibration markings. If visualization of the RV is inadequate, an intravenous contras agent can be administered to obtain better RV border delineation.

The RV shape is complex and its inflow, body and outflow portions cannot all be visualized from one view. Thus imaging of the chamber is necessary from several views. The echocardiographic examination should be performed according to a standard procedure (TABLE I):

**Table 1. Echocardiographic Examination: Methods**

| |
|---|
| 1) Parasternal long axis |
| 2) Parasternal long axis to visualize the tricuspid valve (RV inflow view) |
| 3) Parasternal short axis (multiple levels including the base of heart to visualize RVOT) |
| 4) Apical four-chamber |
| 5) Apical two-chamber (separately of left ventricle and right ventricle) |
| 6) Subcostal long axis |
| 7) Subcostal short axis of RV inflow and outflow |

1) The first echocardiographic window that should be obtained is the **parasternal long axis**. This imaging plane is recorded with the transducer in the third or fourth intercostals space immediate to the left of the sternum. The transducer should be angled so that aortic valve, mitral valve and left ventricle are in their long axis. This view should be performed at a depth that allows visualization of all structures and then at a lower depth focusing on the RV.

Structures of interest in this view include:

- Left ventricle – dimensions and wall motion
- Left atrium – size
- Mitral valve – structure and function
- Aortic valve – structure and function
- Right ventricle – dimension, morphology and wall motion

In this view, M-mode of the LV should be obtained at the highest sweep speed. The line of interrogation should be at the leaflet tip and perpendicular to the long axis of the LV. Color Doppler of the MV and AV should be obtained.

2) The second view is the parasternal long axis of the RV which allows visualization of the tricuspid valve (**RV inflow view**). This is obtained by angling the transducer to the right from the parasternal long axis of the LV and rotating the transducer slightly. The inferoposterior wall of the right ventricular inflow tract under the tricuspid valve is the most important region to be visualized, because it is a frequently affected region. To evaluate this region the transducer should be angled toward the inferior vena cava or the liver. In ARVD this region may appear as thinned and have diastolic bulging or wall motion abnormalities (hypokinesis, akinesis or dyskinesis). In ARVD subjects

the inferoposterior wall motion is generally reduced as compared to healthy subjects. In severe ARVD the only motion in this region is that of the leaflet plane. Color Doppler of the TR jet should also be attempted.

3) The **parasternal short axis** at the aortic valve level is obtained by angling the probe 90° with respect to the parasternal long axis of the LV. This view provides information about the outflow portion of the right ventricle. In many subjects the ratio between the right ventricular outflow tract and the aorta (in systole) will be enlarged. The outflow tract is one of the places where there are saccular dilatations and wall motion abnormalities. The anterior wall, especially in its apical portion, may be commonly affected by fibro-fatty replacement. Therefore, it is important to view the anterior wall of the right ventricle from several short axis views including mid-ventricle and apex. These are obtained by angling or moving the probe more toward the apex while maintaining a tomographic cut of the LV. These views are important for the analysis of the left ventricle and septal configuration.

Color Doppler of pulmonic regurgitation and a peak velocity of the tricuspid regurgitation jet by continuous wave Doppler should be obtained from the short axis views of RV outflow and inflow respectively.

4) The **apical four-chamber** view provides considerable information including the relative sizes of the right and the left ventricle. The four-chamber view is defined as a view which maximizes the LV long axis and the tricuspid and mitral annular dimensions. In this view, the full excursion of the mitral and tricuspid valves should be seen. From this view, the morphology and the motion of the left ventricle and right ventricle are assessed. In order to permit visualization of the trabecular pattern of the RV, an image should be obtained by moving the transducer toward the midline and magnifying the RV. In the apical four chamber view, color Doppler of mitral regurgitation and tricuspid regurgitation should be recorded. Also pulse wave Doppler at the leaflet tips of the mitral and tricuspid valves should be recorded at the fastest sweep speed in order to assess diastolic function. Pulse wave Doppler or a pulmonary vein should be recorded when feasible. Lastly, the continuous wave Doppler of the tricuspid regurgitation jet should be recorded in order to calculate the peak RV systolic pressure.

5) Since the inferoposterior wall of the right ventricle is commonly involved in ARVD, it is important to visualize this region from as many views as possible the **apical RV two-chamber** view. Starting from the apical four-chamber, the transducer is positioned over the RV apex and then angled and rotated to visualize the inferoposterior wall of the RV and its apex. These walls are assessed for wall motion and the myocardial trabecular pattern.

6) The echocardiographic analysis continues with the study of the **subcostal long-axis view**. This view is obtained with the transducer moved to a subxyphoid position and directed superiorly and leftward. The view is aligned so that the orientation of the LV an RV are similar to that obtained in the apical four chamber view. From this subcostal long-axis view one can obtain information about the RV size and motion of its free wall and apex. The transducer is then angled upward to visualize the shape and motion of the RVOT and to assess for saccular dilatation and wall motion abnormalities.

7) Finally the transducer is rotated into the **subcostal short axis view**. From this projection both the inflow tract and the outflow tract of the right ventricle are assessed. Again in this view key findings of ARVD include alteration of motion such as diastolic bulging or wall motion abnormalities of the inflow tract and enlargement, and saccular dilatation of the outflow tract.

The compilation of these views will allow for calculation of:

- Cardiac chamber dimensions (including left ventricle, left atrium, right atrium and right ventricle)
- Right ventricular areas and volumes (RV volume will be calculated by the previously validated biplane area-length method)
- Right ventricular function
    - ♦ Systolic: calculated by "descent of the base" method, endocardial area change method and volume change
    - ♦ Diastolic: E/A wave, deceleration time, dP/dt.
- Right ventricular wall thickness
- Severity of tricuspid valve regurgitation
- Estimation of the right ventricular systolic pressure
- Right ventricular regional function
- Presence and location of RV aneurysms

New echocardiographic perspectives in early diagnozing SCD prone patients

In previous few years we reported of V sign (pic 1,2) as early patognomonic sign in ARVD patients. As for V sign to be searched for we use pulsed wave Doppler tissue imaging in hope to observe an abnormal posterior septal wall motion. The pulsed wave Doppler sample volume (size 4) is usually placed on the right ventricular side at the basal interventricular septum in the apical 4-chamber view, as well as in the long axis parasternal view and in the short axis on the mitral valve level. Special attention is carefully paid to the Doppler velocity to avoid aliasing (Nyquist limit 15cm/s) and aligning the Doppler beam to the interventricular septum to optimize measurements which we obtaine during end expiration. Based on the septal wall motion velocity pattern, peak myocardial velocities are measured in pre-ejection (peak PE), in systole (peak S), in early diastole (peak E) and in late diastole (peak A). Values for all echocardiographic parameters are however, averaged over five cardiac cycles.

It is much easier though, with color coded M mode TDI [3,4,5,6,7,8] to objectivize the diference between normal subject and a patient with ARVD (or any other clinical form above mentioned). Tau point is clearly indicating the region afected with early apoptosis due to any discovered defect in cell to cell athesion proteins that loose contact as a consequence of diferent forces applied to he locus minoris resistentiae in the double helicoid structure of the heart.

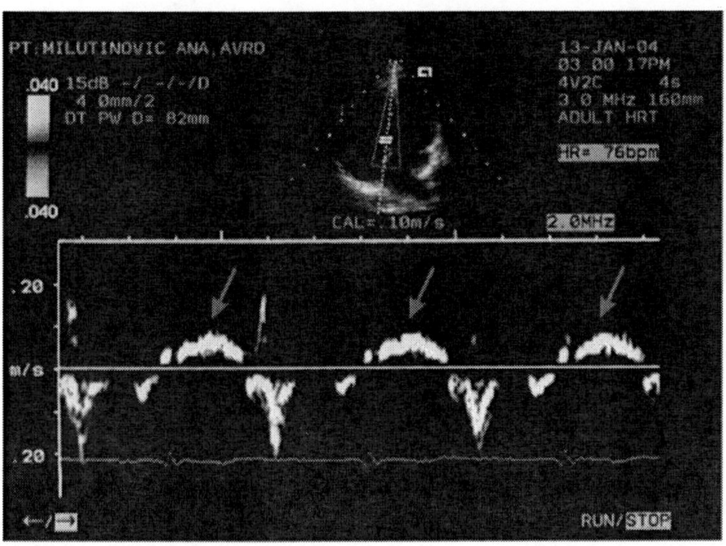


Figure 1. ARVD pt. Red arrow depicits V sign postsystolic shortening.

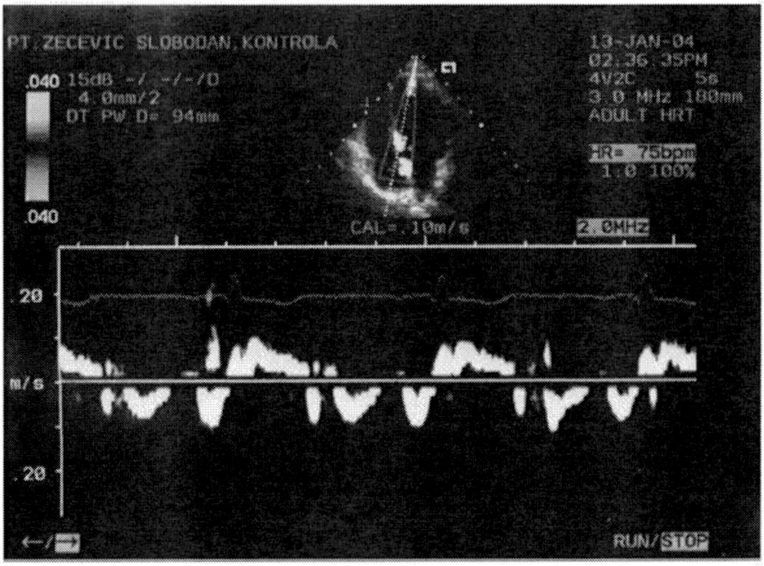


Figure 2. Normal individual. Postsystolic lenthening- no V sign.

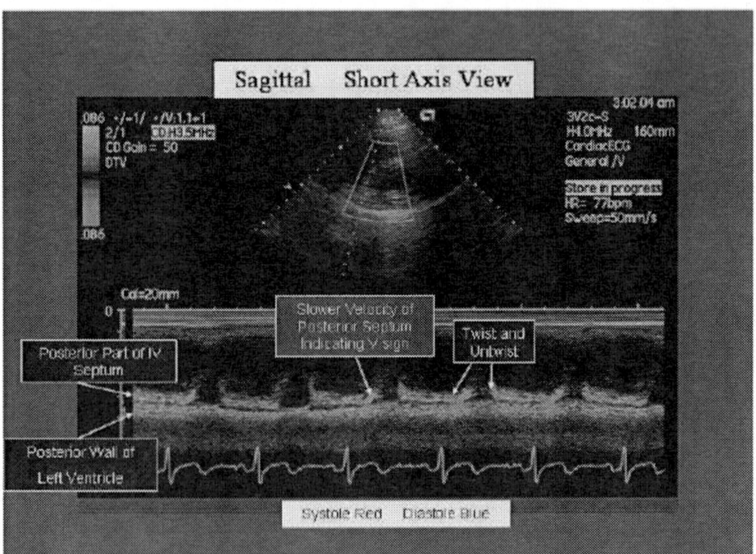


Figure 3. ARVD pt. Note the existence of V sign.

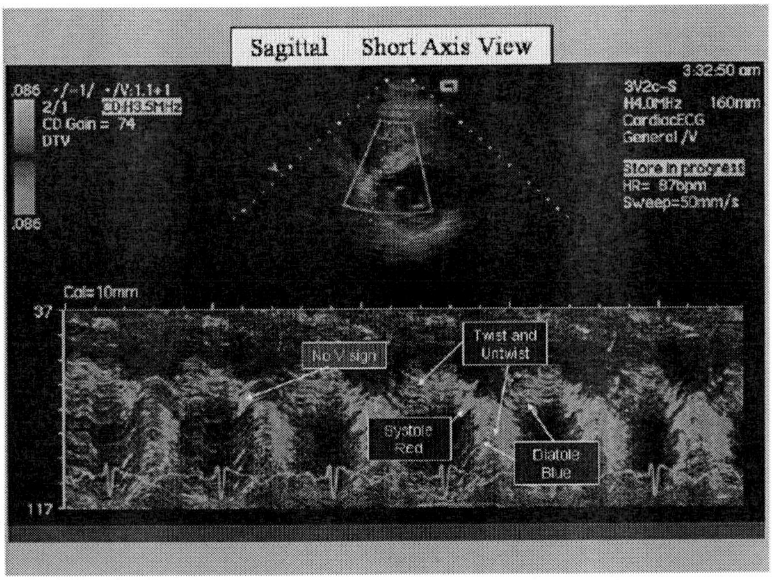


Figure 4. Normal individual-no V sign.

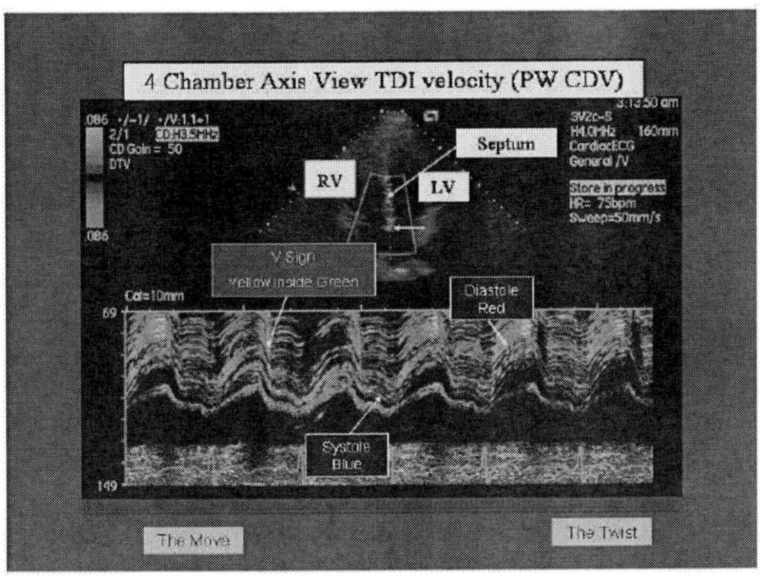


Figure 5. ARVD pt. Note the existence of V sign.

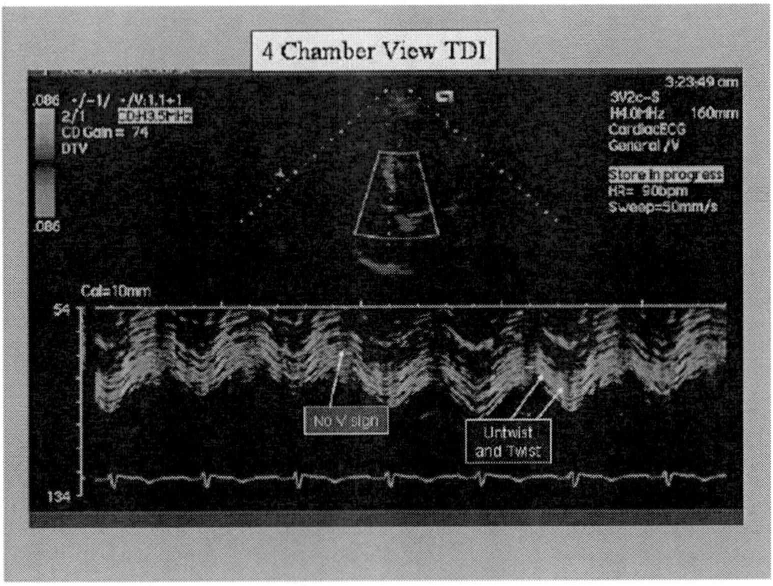


Figure 6. Normal individual-no V sign.

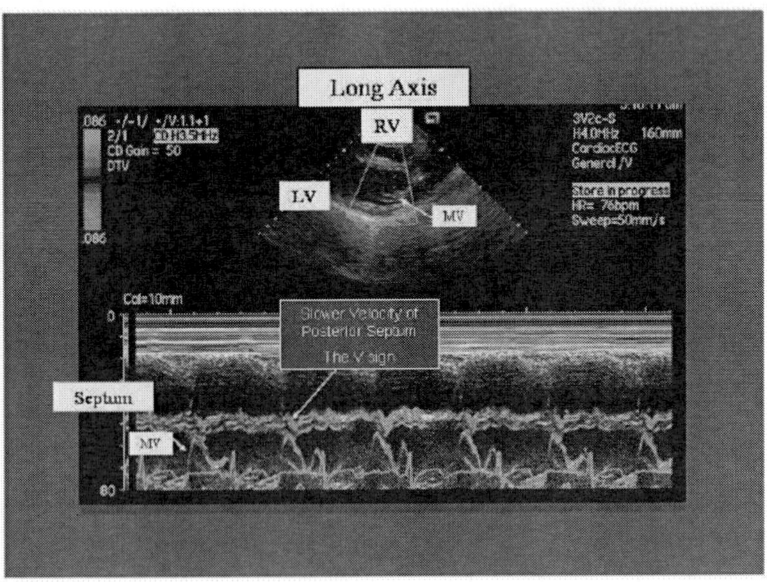


Figure 7. ARVD pt. Note the existence of V sign.

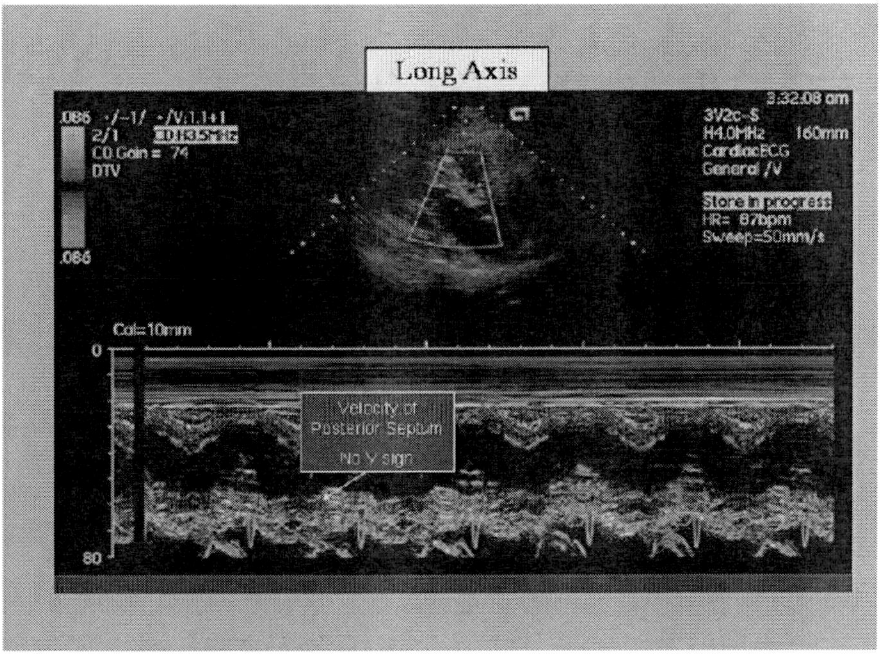


Figure 8. Normal individual-no V sign.

However, in our 10 year experience with patients with ARVD, a second sign in close relation to the existence of Tau point has been discovered and named "T sign". This sign is also pathognomonic of ARVD in relation to registered changes in motion of the septal cusp of tricuspid valve at the early stage of the disease. The explaination for this lies in the affected region of the Tau point where the loss of support for the posterior part of cusp exists. In search for this T sign echo examination is performed in similar fashion. 2D echo is always performed in apical four chamber view with technique of pulsed Doppler tissue imaging. The pulsed wave Doppler sample volume (size 4) is to be placed on the right ventricular side at the basal part of septal cusp and special attention paid to aligning the Doppler beam to the interventricular septum to optimize measurements which are obtained during end expiration. Consequently transtricuspid flow profile is being recorded and values of all echocardiographic parameters are averaged over five cardiac cycles to avoid respiratory changes. 2D echo examination is to be performed in each patient in apical 4-chamber view, parasternal long axis view and parasternal short axis view on the mitral valve area level.

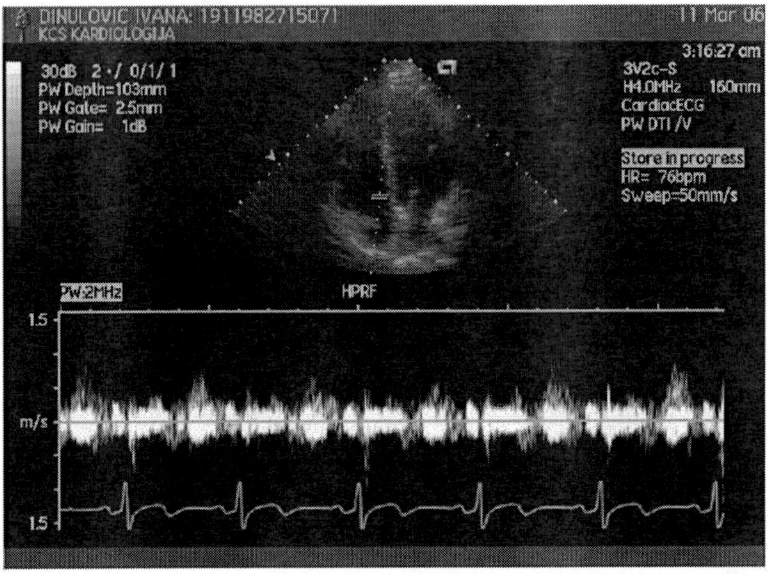


Figure 9. Characteristic appearance of E/A ratio changeable interplay.

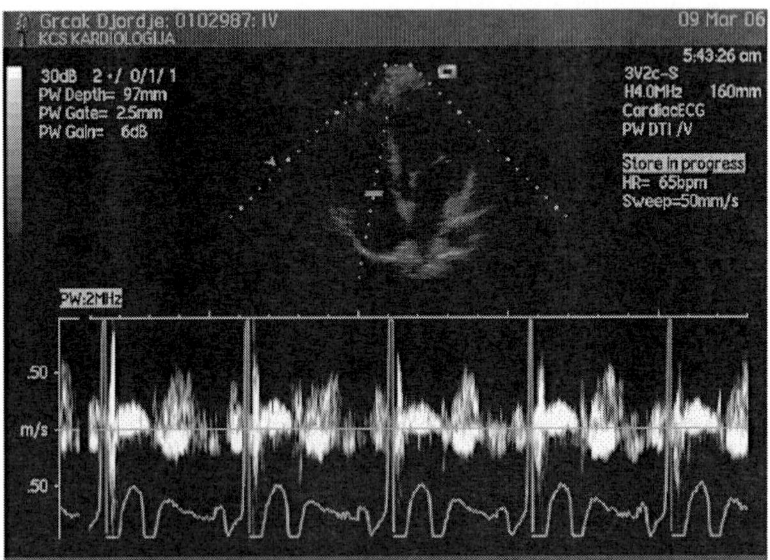


Figure 10. Normal transtricuspid flow-slight changes in E amplitude due to respiratory changes.

Significant change in E/A velocity due to complex volume oscillations in right heart as a consequence of septal cusp lack of support in the posterior basal part due to existence of Tau point in pts prone to SCD. E wave velocity measures 0.5; 0.7; 0.6; 0.4; 0.5; 0.8. A wave measures 0.3; 0.2; 0.4; 0.4; 0.5; 0.1. It means the more blood is hold in the right atrium the more has to be pulled out in the next consecutive beat (pic 9).

Conversely, in normal subjects there is only respiratory pressure volume changes in empting RV (pic 10). It is therefore possible, if no other arrhythmia exists to spot this sophisticated interdependent relationship that is clearly visible in ARVD or any other form SCD risk patients even in the very early phase of the disease process, long ago any morphological changes in the heart may occur.

## ECG Newly Observed Signs

Among research attempts in discovering new diagnostic signs in ARVD patients Dr Guy Fontaine has reported of late potentials derived epsilon waves in diferent localization on ECG and named them prepsilon, topsilon, bipsilon, tripsilon, and giant epsilon during last Cardiostim conference. This idea is not easily aplicable because of technical limitations and quality of ECG machine but it is of significant importance in the clinical practice.

## Vectorcardiography in Diagnosing ARVD

However, in evaluating ECG tracings vectorcardiography is more susceptible to delicate changes and is more superior than late potentials (signal averaged electrocardiograms) in detecting electricaly non conductive areas of myocardium. In that sense Dr Ivana Vranic has reported of specific early changes due to Tau point. The explaination of this lies in the electrical propagation through HVMB and vector sequence by time changeble. It is now subject of ongoing trial in checking its wide aplicability.

## Discussion

Discovery of the ventricular myocardial band by Dr Francisco Torrent Guasp reconciled form and function of ventricular myocardium, giving explaination for electrical and mechanical events in human heart. It has been clearly demonstrated by fast Fourier analyses of ventricular MUGA scans, that muscular contractile activity, during the cardiac cycle, progresses (in a peristaltoid manner), along successive VMB segments. Since the excitation necessarily precedes contraction, the most logical pattern of ventricular electrical activation should follow both spatially and temporarily, previously described sequence of its mechanical action. V sign is therefore easy to explain because crista supraventricularis is driven by three orthogonaly opposed forces as embaded in inferioposterior septal part being ephemerally behind the time in the contraction. The observation of septal posterior displacement by 2D echo may be in accordance with localized cell to cell adhesion protein distortion suspected in this condition, or localized apoptosis demonstrated in the posteroseptal part of crista supraventricularis by Dr Thomas N. James. On the basis of anatomic study of human and other mammalian hearts, it has been suggested that it is crucial to the understanding of right ventricular failure to consider the normal functions of the crista supraventricularis. As long as the crista supraventricularis remains intact, left ventricular systole can tether even the damaged right ventricular free wall sufficiently to empty the right ventricle into the pulmonary artery. An intact crista supraventricularis is also necessary for normal function of the tricuspid valve, both by its purse-string action on the tricuspid orifice and by providing essential support for the anterior leaflet of the tricuspid valve. For its optimal mechanical effectiveness in coordinating and facilitating hemodynamic efficiency of the right ventricle with that of the left ventricle (including most of the interventricular septum), the anatomic configuration of the apoptotic tissue (septal band of the crista supraventricularis) in the upper right side of the crest of the interventricular septum explains some probable contractile advantages. Although the connection of the septal band with the rest of the crista supraventricularis is thin when seen in cross section, it is actually a broad sheet extending from an area posterior to the membranous interventricular septum to a region well anterior to the normal location of the His bundle. Furthermore, the bottom of the septal band tissue seen in cross section has a pronglike configuration, suggesting a firm anchor deep within the mass of interventricular septal myocardium.

## CONCLUSION

Because right ventricular function may be impared either by primary right sided heart disease, or secondary to left sided cardiomyopathy or valvular heart disease it is obvious that RV function should be evaluated with caution. In practice, clinicians largely rely on non-invasive imaging methods for assessment of RV function. Two dimensional echocardiography is the mainstay for analysis of RV function, but recently alternative techniques have been proposed, including tissue Doppler imaging (TDI) techniques, three dimensional echocardiography, magnetic resonance imaging (MRI), and even invasive assessment of pressure-volume loops. Also, vectorcardiography gives clear cut potential in analyzing RV function and even eary diagnosis for the risk of SCD due to inhereted disorders that affect desmosomes, such as ARVD as most common one.

Valid WHO criteria during last 12 years failed to detect disease at its early stage and recommended diagnostic methods were shown to have low sensitivity for majority of patients even in its overt phase (because of lack of scoring system). Investigation of this population is further complicated by disease rarity and lack of large databases. New research published data give priority to vectorcardiography and ultrasound.

The possible explanation for this lies in the existence of specific place in the heart exposed to most physical forces during cardiac cycle. Nevertheless, this place is *locus minoris rezistentio* during contraction and relaxation of the heart. It is presently focus of ongoing clinical study regarding two aforementioned methods in detecting early stage of ARVD/C. It is also registered by WIPO as SOPHIE methodology (suggesting wisdom to detect). Soon enough we can expect this technique to be incorporated in newly medical equipment (for stratification of risk for SCD).

## REFERENCES

[1] Myerburg RJ, Castellanos A. Cardiac arest and sudden death. In: Zipes DP, Libby P, Bonow RO and Braunwald E, ed. Braunwald's *Heart Disease: A Textbook of Cardiovascular Medicine. 7th edn. Elsevier Saunders Company,* Philadelphia, PA, 2004:865-908.

[2] Priori SG, Aliot E, Blomstrom-Lundqvist C et al. Task force on sudden cardiac death of the European Society of Cardiology. *Eur. Heart J.* 2001; 22: 1374-1450.

[3] Escobedo LG, Zack MM: Comparison of sudden and nonsudden coronary deaths in the United States. *Circulation.* 1996; 93: 2033-36.

[4] Arntz HR, Willich SN et al. Diurnal, weekly and seasonal variation of sudden death. Population based analysis of 24 061 consecutive cases. *Eur. Heart J.* 2000; 21:315-20.

[5] Holmberg M, Holmberg S, Herlitz J. Incidence, duration and survival of ventricular fibrilation in out-of-hospital cardiac arrest patients in Sweden. *Resuscitation.* 2000; 44:7-17.

[6] Rampazzo A., Nava A., Danieli G.A., Buja G. et al. The gene for arrhythmogenic right ventricular cardiomyopathy maps to chromosome 14q23-q24, 1994, *Hum. Moll. Gen.* 3, No 6959-962

[7] Fukushima Y., Byers,M.G., Watkins P.C. et al.(1990) *Cytogenet. Cell. Genet.,* 53,232-233

[8] Lansman J.B., Franco A.Jr.(1991) *J. Muscle. Res. Cell. Motil.,* 12,409-411

[9] Saffitz E. Jeffrey. 2005. Dependence of Electrical Coupling on Mechanical Coupling in Cardiac Myocites. *Ann. N. Y. Sci.* 1047.336.-344.

[10] Fatkin, D.and R..M.Graham. 2002. Molecular mechanisms of inherited cardiomyopathies. *Physiol. Rev.* 82. 945-980.

[11] McKoy, G.,N.Protonotarios,A. Crosby,et al.2000.Identification of a deletionof plakoglobin in arrhythmogenic right ventricular cardiomyopathy with palmoplantar keratoderma and wooly hair-Naxos disease. *Lancet.* 355. 2119-2124.

[12] Fisher SA, Langille LB, Srivastava D. Apoptosis during cardiovascular development. 2000. *Circulation Research.* November 10, 856-64.

[13] Perlman H, Maillard L, Krasinski K et al. Evidence for the rapid onset of apoptosis in medial smooth muscle cells after baloon injury. *Circulation.* 1997; 95:981-7.

[14] Ashkenazi A, Dixit V. Death receptors: signalling and modulation. *Science.* 1998; 281: 1305-8.

[15] Torrent-Guasp F,Buckberg GD,Clemente C,Cox JL et al "The structure and function of the helical heart and its buttress wrapping.I.The normal macroscopic structure of the heart.. Semin Thorac. Cardiovasc. Surg. 2001;13(4):301-19

[16] Torrent-Guasp F,Kocica MJ,Corno A,Komeda M et al."Systolic ventricular filling. *Eur. J. Cardiothorac. Surg.* 2004;25(3):376-86

[17] Lunkenheimer PP,Redmann K,Florek J,Fassancht U .et al "The forces generated within the musculature of the left ventricular wall. *Heart.* 2004;90:200-7

[18] Streeter DD,Torrent -Guasp F.Geodesic paths in the left ventricle of the mammalian heart. *Circualation.* 1973;48 (Suppl. 4):4-14.

[19] Greenbaum RA, Ho SY, GibsonDG ,Becker AE, Anderson RH.Left ventricular fibre architecture in man. *British Heart Journal.* 1981; 45:248-63

[20] Buckberg GD, Clemente C,Cox JL, Coghlan HC, Castella M, Torrent-Guasp F et al.The structure and the function of the helical heart and its buttress wrapping IV.Concepts of dynamic function from the nirmal macroscopic helical structure. *Semin Thoracic Cardiovasc. Surg*. 2001; 13(4):342-57

[21] Torrent- Guasp F,Ballerter M, Buckberg GD et al.Spatial orientation of the ventricular muscle band:physiologic contribution and surgical implicamions. *J. Thorac. Cardiovasc. Surg*. 2001;122(2):389-92

[22] Marino B, Corno AF. Spiral pattern: universe, normal heart, and complex congenital defects. *J. Thorac. Cardiovasc. Surg.* 2003;126(4) 1225-6.

[23] Ivana Vranic. Un nouveau signe echocardiographique pour identifier la DVDA. *Cardinale* Tome XVI No 2 Fevrier 2004, p 22-4.

[24] McKenna WJ, Thiene G et al Diagnosis of arrhythmogenic right ventricular dysplasia/cardiomyopathy. Task Force of the Working Group Myocardial and Pericardial Disease of the European Society of Cardiology and of the Scientific Council on Cardiomyopathies of the International Society and Federation of Cardiology. *Br. Heart J.* 1994 Mar;71(3):215-8.

[25] Thiene G, Nava A et al. Right ventricular cardiomyopathy and sudden death in young people. *N. Engl. J. Med.* 1988 Jan 21;318(3):129-33.

[26] Fontaine G, Fontaliran F, Frank R. Arrhythmogenic right ventricular cardiomyopathies: clinical forms and main differential diagnoses. *Circulation.* 1998 Apr 28;97(16):1532-5.

[27] Corrado D, Fontaine G et al. Arrhythmogenic right ventricular dysplasia/cardiomyopathy: need for an international registry. Study Group on Arrhythmogenic Right Ventricular Dysplasia/Cardiomyopathy of the Working Groups on Myocardial and Pericardial Disease and Arrhythmias of the European Society of Cardiology and of the Scientific Council on Cardiomyopathies of the World Heart Federation. *Circulation.* 2000 Mar 21;101(11):E101-6.

[28] Yoerger DM, Marcus F, Sherrill D, et al. For the Multidisciplinary Study of Right Ventricular Dysplasia. Echocardiographic findings in patients meeting task force criteria for arrhythmogenic right ventricular dysplasia: new insights from the Multidisciplinary Study of Right Ventricular Dysplasia. *J. Am. Coll. Cardiol.* 2005;45:860 –5.

[29] Ivana I Vranic. Assessment of right ventricular function in ARVC/D patients by 2D ECHO. Abstracts of EUROECHO 7 December 3-6, 2003. *Eur. J. Echocard.* 2003, Vol 4 Suppl 1, p S74

[30] Ivana I Vranic. Pathognomonic sign of ARVC/D by Echo? Abstracts of EUROECHO 7 December 3-6, 2003. *Eur. J. Echocard.* 2003, Vol 4 Suppl 1, p S74

[31] Ivana I Vranic, M Ristic, T Simic. Specific and sensitive enough to reveal the fruste forms of arrhythmogenic right ventricular dysplasia. *J. Am. Soc. Echocardiog.* May 2004, Vol 17 No 5: 524.

[32] Ivana I Vranic, M Ristic et al.. Septal cusp irregular motion of tricuspid valve in ARVD patients. *Echocardiog.* May 2004, Vol 21 No 4: 358.

[33] Ivana I Vranic, T Simic. Contribution of the crista supraventricularis function in development of heart failure in ARVD patients. *Eur. J. Echocardiog.* Dec 2004, Vol 5 Suppl 1:177S.

[34] Ivana I Vranic, M Matic. Sudden cardiac death in young athletes- is it preventable? *Europace.* June 2005, Vol 7 -Suppl 1: 85.

[35] Ivana I Vranic, Mihailo Matić. Arrhythmogenic right ventricular dysplasia non qualifying for criteria of WHF but echo positive. *Eur. J. Echocardiog.* Dec 2005, Vol 6 Suppl 1:S26.

[36] Ivana I Vranic. Another pathognomonic sign in arrhythmogenic right ventricular dysplasia vizualized by pulsed wave doppler in septal cusp of tricuspid valve. *J. Am. Soc. Echocardiog*. May 2006, Vol 19 No 5: 632.

# INDEX

## D

## E

## H



## I

## J



## K



## L

## M



## N

## O



## P

## S

## T